MASTER THE ART OF

AGING
GRACEFULLY

Power Up Your Youthfulness, Apply Smart Skills,
Build Financial Stability And Grow Old Mindfully

VIKRAM KHAITAN

PUBLISHED BY:

VIKRAM KHAITAN

(vikram.khaitan@gmail.com)

ISBN-13:   9798599746904

ASIN:

COPYRIGHT © Vikram Khaitan 2021

All rights reserved. No parts of this publication may be reproduced, stored, retrieved, printed, and transmitted, in any form or by any means, electronic, mechanical, photocopying, recording, or otherwise, without the express prior permission of the author.

TABLE OF CONTENTS

INTRODUCTION 4
Part 1: Health, Happiness and Life! 12
Chapter 1: HEALTH & YOUTHFULNESS 13
Chapter 2: BE A HAPPY SOUL 34
Chapter 3: STAY ACTIVE & AGILE 52
Part 2: Financial Independence 63
Chapter 4: BE FINANCIALLY WISE 64
Part 3: Safety and Security 72
Chapter 5: SAFETY AT HOME 73
Chapter 6: SAFETY OUTSIDE HOME 78
Chapter 7: TRAVEL SAFE 81
Chapter 8: CYBER SECURITY 85
Part 4: Aging Gracefully 88
Chapter 9: REVERSE AGING 89
Chapter 10: THE SECRET OF JAPANESE LONGEVITY
.... 101
Chapter 11: AGE-ing To SAGE-ing 105
Chapter 12: The Conclusion 114
ONE MOMENT PLEASE 120
GRATITUDE 121
ABOUT THE AUTHOR 122
DISCLAIMER 123
MY PREVIOUS WORKS 124
REFERENCES 129

INTRODUCTION

"There is a fountain of youth: It is your mind, your talents, the creativity you bring to your life and the lives of people you love. When you learn to tap this source, you will truly have defeated age."— Sophia Loren [Actor]

What is the sunset in life?

As the Sun rises every morning and sets in the evening, it sends a reminder to all of us that there is just one thing in this universe that happens most silently yet incessantly. This one thing is aging of every living being with passaging time. Everyone becomes older by the minute, yet yearns to remain youthful forever. With the accumulation of experiences of life and a collection of memories, the human mind develops a golden radiance. That's why the sunset years are called golden years. People react to similar situations differently. Could there be a shift in paradigm by wishing for a golden sunset instead of remaining averse to the inevitable?

How important is youthfulness?

As age advances every moment and you see that becoming old is inevitable, how important is it to keep your youthfulness?

Do you ever wish you could stay young forever? Or is it really worth it?

Medical advancement and modern sciences have made it possible to increase the life expectancy rate. The average life expectancy rate in the year 1900 was around 40 years and in 2020 it is over 72.6 years. This means that humans nowadays are living one and a half times longer than their ancestors lived a century ago.

It is a constant human endeavor to strive for living longer. Even the blessings get imbibed by this desire. "Long live the queen!"

Do you want to say goodbye to ageing?

Israeli scientists are close to reverse ageing by 25 years. Israeli scientists have carried out research that will help fight ageing. They conducted the research on 35 volunteers who were over 64 years of age.

They provided the volunteers with clean oxygen for 90 minutes a day, five days a week in a pressurized chamber. The experiment continued for three months and the result was appalling.

The scientists claim that ageing in all 35 volunteers got arrested, which means the researches in a period of just three months successfully carried out the process of reverse ageing.

India is a land of mysticism and philosophy which holds the answer to every problem and the world is gradually recognizing the values in its rich and ancient philosophies. Join me for a brief journey into the past through a story that reflects man's desire for longevity. This is the history of several centuries ago.

YAYATI was the son of Nahusha, the great Chandravanshi king who once presided as Indra in heaven. He was a famous ruler who kept his kin happy. He had two ravishingly beautiful women in his life. Devayani (his wife) was the daughter of the asura Guru Shukracharya. Sharmishtha (his mistress), the daughter of the asura ruler, Vrushaparva. Yayati got extremely enamored with Sharmishtha, while he was very little attracted to Devayani.

His lust for Sharmishtha lands him into a situation where he got cursed with old age. However, it eventually turns out to be a boon with 1,000 years of youth, and he gains knowledge equal to the supreme God himself.

After losing his youth because of a revile from sage Shukracharya, he gave Yayati the concession of having the option to trade his old age with a willing child of his. His two sons from Devayani, Yadu and Turvasu, declined the offer right away.

The initial two children from Sharmishtha excessively would not give their youth to their father. It is just the last son Puru from Sharmishta, who concurs. Yayati along these lines declares Puru should be the inheritor of his realm and wealth. The price Puru pays for this, is bearing 1,000 years of old age.

Yayati enjoys carnal desires for 1,000 years of youth. Yayāti appreciates all the joys of the senses for a very long time. By experiencing joys without limit, he comes to understand its absolute uselessness, saying: "Know this beyond any doubt... not all the food, abundance and women of the world can satiate the desire of a solitary man of uncontrolled desires. Longing for sensual pleasures never extinguishes, yet exasperated by extravagance even as ghee when poured into fire expands it. One who aspires to peace and happiness should instantly renounce craving and seek instead, that which neither grows old, nor ceases - no matter how old the body may become."

Having discovered astuteness by following the streets of abundance, Yayāti thankfully restores the youth of his son Puru and reclaims his old age. When Yayati acknowledges his old age once more, Puru turns into the primary ruler of what we might know as the Pourava lineage, precursors to kings, for example, Dushyanta, Bharata, and the later Kauravas and Pandavas.

Yayati repudiated the world to spend his leftover days as an ascetic in the forest. His profound practices are, finally, honored with progress and, alone in the profound forests, the Gods compensate him with rising to 'swarga' - the radiant domain of the upright, controlled by Indra, that is just one stage underneath the definitive freedom of moksha.

A case for longevity vs purposeful life

"Ageing is an extraordinary process where you become the person you always should have been."—David Bowie [Singer, Lyricist]

The pursuit of medical science vs the story of Yayati is paradoxical. It took Yayati 1000 years to realize the importance of respecting the natural cycle of birth and death. It might take 100 or more years for the medical science to discover that the magnanimity of scientific research is not into preserving life into an old and disabled body. Medical science and life's health practices have to ensure that it must yield solutions to keep the youthfulness of the body and the mind. An extended life-span should not become a predicament in disguise to drag an old and invalid body. It should enable the people on this planet to live a meaningful and healthy life which offers reasons enough to celebrate life itself.

Stories from the past are pedagogical. They were well-researched philosophies of their times, that were told to the common folks through the medium of story-telling.

Besides philosophy and medicine, there is a point of view from economics as well. The first wave of industrialized and well-developed nations like Japan and U.K. now have a majority of their population comprising old people. India has two-thirds of their population aged under 35 years. The middle East has a significantly large population in their teens. This means that nature shall burden the countries that have a youthful demography today with older people in the times to come. Eldercare shall be the business for tomorrow, but what about productivity and usefulness of these people? Will they live a longer part of their lives with youthful exuberance, or will they drag themselves through the pains and miseries of old age with a delayed respite? Also, if there are many people living a longer phase of youth, the population will expand rapidly and cause a scarcity of resources even further. Take a case that the normal retirement age extends by five more years, the young would have to wait longer to get into a job until the older ones have vacated. Hence there needs to be a balance between everything as the humans live longer with scientific development.

Ageing vs Maturity

"Growing old is mandatory, but growing up is optional."—Chili Davis, [Baseball player and current coach]

At the cellular level, millions of body cells die every day and as many are born as well. During the growing age, more cells are born than those die every day, hence one grows. The reverse happens after 30. It does not regenerate as many cells after 30 as they die. That's what we know as growing old.

Growing up does not tie to the chronological age. Some people grow old inevitably beyond their 90s, yet they lack basic maturity while there are quite young people who gain mental and spiritual maturity at an early age. Swami Vivekananda led a group of spiritualists in his late 20s.

Sometimes younger people get brought up around adults, especially if they are the firstborn. They learn to talk like adults. They also understand their younger siblings better and hence gain to be adept in communicating with the young and old alike.

Some children display a wide range of sensitivity and sensibility to the environment they grow in. They don't learn the same way as other children who are less sensitive to the environment. To be mature, one must learn from experiences in life rather than just gaining knowledge.

Some people accept responsibilities much too young and don't get to act like children. The school of hard knocks forces maturity on them before they can cope with. Young adults can choose maturity, leave home, to figure out how to earn their loaf of bread, accept adult responsibilities, while others of their age are still children.

Maturity is understanding of the world and your relationship with it. Initially, children don't understand the world, but they do observe cause and effect of behaviors of those around, and it is those behaviors they imitate to know how others react to them.

What happens when you are more matured from an early age? You develop more patience to deal with people, but you become less affected by them. It immerses you in your passions, and you find it easier to remove yourself from situations. You do your job as a person who conveys the blessings from the universe to the benefactor, and then you leave. Your mind has convinced you don't need people, but in reality, we all do.

Maturity is a state of mind when an individual can realize what is happening around him/her, to understand the rationale behind those happenings and does not get too elated nor too depressed by outcome. Thus he/she can absorb pressures and remain unperturbed by the surrounding situations.

Why this book?

"There are six myths about old age: 1. That it's a disease, a disaster. 2. That we are mindless. 3. That we are sexless. 4. That we are useless. 5. That we are powerless. 6. That we are all alike." — Maggie Kuhn [Ageism Activist]

The youth of today have to expect what holds for them in the future and prepare themselves to face the world tomorrow with more resourcefulness and confidence. What can they do today to ensure a better tomorrow? How can they invest into a sunshine future for a golden sunset?

This book is for the youth to learn how to use the philosophies of life in tandem with the gifts of modern medical science, to learn how to preserve their youth and conserve their energy and resources as they grow older every day.

As a young person, while reading this book, you will discover how to power up your youthfulness through investing in health, happiness, relationships, safety, security and gain wisdom for ageing gracefully.

"Despise not growing old…it is a privilege which many are denied."

Part 1: Health, Happiness and Life!

Chapter 1: HEALTH & YOUTHFULNESS

"Health is a state of complete harmony of the body, mind and spirit. When one is free from physical disabilities and mental distractions, the gates of the soul open?"—B.K.S. Iyengar [Yoga teacher]

According to the World Health Organization (W.H.O.), common conditions in older age include hearing loss, cataracts and refractive errors, back and neck pain and osteoarthritis, chronic obstructive pulmonary disease, diabetes, depression, and dementia. As people age, they are more likely to experience several conditions at the same time.

It also characterizes older age by the emergence of several complex health states that occur only later in life and that do not fall into discrete disease categories. We commonly call these **geriatric syndromes**. They are often the consequence of multiple underlying factors and include frailty, urinary incontinence, falls, delirium, blood pressure and ulcers.

Under a recent W.H.O. Resolution (67/13), a comprehensive *Global Strategy and Action Plan on Ageing and Health* is being developed by W.H.O. in consultation with member states and other partners. The strategy and action plan draws on the evidence of the World report on ageing and health and builds on existing activities to address 5 priority areas for action.

1. **Commitment to Healthy Ageing.** Requires awareness of the value of Healthy Ageing and sustained commitment and action to plan evidence-based policies that strengthen the abilities of older persons.

2. **Aligning health systems with the needs of older populations.** Health systems need to get better organized around older people's needs and preferences, designed to enhance older people's intrinsic capacity, and integrated across settings and care providers.

3. **Developing systems for providing long-term care.** Systems of long-term care are required in all countries to meet the needs of older people. This requires developing, sometimes from nothing, governance systems, infrastructure and workforce capacity.

4. **Creating age-friendly environments.** This will require actions to combat ageism, enable autonomy and support Healthy Ageing in all policies and at all levels of government.

5. **Improving measurement, monitoring and understanding.** Focused research, new metrics and analytical methods are needed for a wide range of ageing issues. This work builds on

the extensive work W.H.O. has done in improving health statistics and information, for example through the W.H.O. Study on Global AGEing and adult health (SAGE).

Immunization and Immunity

"I believe the best way to activate genius within the immune system is by ingesting certain superherbs and superfoods, taking probiotics and cultured foods, minimizing toxic food exposure by eating pure organic raw-living foods, and making appropriate healthy lifestyle improvements." - David Wolfe [Raw food advocate]

I remember those dreadful mass inoculation days when I was in school. Firstly. The school would keep that date a secret and second, they would announce some exam on that day to ensure maximum attendance. Anybody trying to hide beneath the tables would get snuffed out and inoculated. They placed a drop of antigen on the arm and stabbed a needle point several times to penetrate the subcutaneous vaccine. Things have changed a lot since then. Now every newborn gets an immunization card with a pre-scheduled calendar for vaccines. You can add in that, the other vaccinations that get invented over time. All other animals, besides humans, are subject to the rule of "survival of the fittest" where the weak perish and the strong survive to procreate. This way nature filters away many anomalies in their genealogy. For humans, their foremost responsibility is to work upon their immunity. Beginning with immunization, one can boost one's immunity through other means as well such as regulation of diet, supplements, exercise, mindfulness and yoga.

Here are 9 natural ways to improve your immunity.

1. Get some excellent quality of sleep–it links inadequate sleep to higher susceptibility to illness. Adults should aim to get 6 or more hours of sleep each night, while teens need 7–9 hours and younger children and infants up to 12-14 hours. Getting adequate rest may strengthen your natural immunity. Try limiting screen time for an hour before bed, as the blue light emitted from your phone, TV, and computer may disrupt your circadian rhythm, or your body's natural wake-sleep cycle.

2. Eat more whole plant food - Foods like fruits, vegetables, nuts, seeds, and legumes are rich in nutrients and antioxidants that may give you an upper hand against harmful pathogens. The antioxidants in these foods help decrease inflammation by combatting unstable compounds called free radicals, which can cause inflammation when they build up in your body in high levels. Vow to shun processed food like refined flours, oils, fried, baked, cheesy, sugary and too much salted foods.

3. Healthy fats are good - Healthy fats, like cow milk ghee (clarified butter) and those found in cold pressed olive oil, mustard oil and salmon, may boost your body's immune response to pathogens by decreasing inflammation.

4. Take probiotics to improve gut bacteria - Fermented foods are rich in beneficial bacteria called probiotics, which populate your digestive tract. These foods include milk curds, yogurt, dosa, idli, khamiri roti, sauerkraut, kimchi, kefir, and natto and some home brewed fermented drinks like kanji, sake and grape wine.

5. Cut down on whites—As a kid, I always got reminded that things good for the health are often bland or insipid, while most delectable cuisines are bad for health. However, it is wise to cut down on white foods like salt, sugar, refined flour and dairy products.

6. Drink water—Stay hydrated with water. I consider a glassful an hour during your wake time as a good intake. Do not substitute your water intake with soda, tea or coffee because they are diuretic. Diuretic substances make you urinate frequently, resulting into water loss. Regular water intake helps you to detoxify at the cellular level. Munching juicy salads like cucumber and lettuce help in water retention during scorching summer.

7. Regular moderate exercise - Although prolonged intense exercise can suppress your immune system, moderate exercise can give it a boost. A brisk walk routine, yoga, or light sports like tennis, badminton, table tennis, squash, swimming, etc are very good habits to keep.

8. Manage your stress level - Relieving stress and anxiety is key to immune health. Long-term stress promotes inflammation, and imbalances in immune cell function. Stress causes maximum damage to health. During a stressful episode, the body produces toxins that can cause severe damage to organs and even produce carcinogenic risk at the cellular level.

9. Intimacy - Intimacy with the spouse enhances emotional well-being, relaxes, decreases stress, and makes us feel great. A study conducted by Psychology Today magazine found that the more active and satisfying a person's intimacy is, the fitter and healthier they are. Look forward to it and try to make it happen as frequently as possible.

Periodic Health Check

The best time to visit a doctor is when you are not suffering from an acute illness. That's the time you can have a periodic health check done to rule out the onset of any disease. Once in six months is ideal, but once in a year is a must. Besides the blood work, get your eyes, ears, dental and Ortho check-ups done as well. Skin care is also very essential because it is the first to give away your age.

Your periodic blood work scans your haemogram i.e. the basic elements of blood constitution, the Lipid profile (heart), Renal profile (Kidney function), Liver profile, Thyroid profile, Diabetes profile and Vitamin deficiencies. Different medical centers may have variable test packages.

It is good to have a trustworthy general physician (GP) as your family doctor instead of walking into a super specialist. The GP shall examine your health check reports along with your vitals and guide you for further treatment if required. In the third world countries there is an absence of two-tier consultation. People often skip the GP and directly go from one super specialist to the other.

Eye care

Changes in vision is often the first undeniable sign of ageing.

- The lens stiffens, making focusing on close objects harder.
- The lens becomes denser, making seeing in the dim light harder.
- The pupil reacts more slowly to changes in light hence it takes time for the vison to re-adjust with change in illumination.

- The lens yellows, changing the way we perceive colors.
- The number of nerve cells decrease, impairing depth perception.
- The eyes produce less fluid, making them feel dry.

There are two compulsory precautions every day.

(1) Splash the eyes twice a day with cold water and (2) never rub the eyes for any reason.

Visit the ophthalmologist at least twice a year for a routine check-up.

Ear care

Most changes in hearing are probably due as much to noise exposure as to ageing. Exposure to loud noise over time damages the ear's ability to hear. Some changes in hearing occur as people age, regardless of their exposure to loud noise. As people age, hearing high-pitched sounds becomes more difficult. We consider this change as age-associated hearing loss.

Avoid earphone, wireless ear pods, loud music or loud noise at work place because these would impair your hearing ability at an early age. Never poke ear buds or objects into the ear. Visit the ear doctor once in six months, or at least once a year.

Dental care

Cavities, tooth decay, gum recession, bad breath and other oral problems are common with ageing.

Brush your teeth twice every day, once in the morning and once before sleep. Flossing between the teeth is more important than brushing. Use a scraper to keep the tongue clean. Rub your upper cleft with your thumb while rinsing. Rinse your mouth every time after you eat or drink something. Do not brush too frequently, as it might scrub away the tooth enamel. Mouth-wash solutions are too acidic and not too good for regular use. Do not clench or grind your teeth for no reason. You can easily ruin your teeth with smoking, chewing tobacco, beetle-nuts, sugar candies etc. Munching on sugar free chewing gum is a healthy habit.

Ortho care

Bone degeneration, erosion of cartilage, falls and fractures, osteoporosis (porosity of bones because of calcium deficiency) are common problems with ageing. Do not start jogging at a later age if you are not into sports. Do not undergo heavy exercise and squatting if you are not used to it since childhood.

Right postures, moderate exercise, calcium rich food, vitamin D, collagen supplements, are good for bones. Go for a bone density test and a general check-up once in two years after you are 50.

Brain care

Number of brain cells and neurotransmitters decrease with age, and the blood flow gets reduced as well. It hampers the cognitive abilities and impairs the reflexes. Alzheimer's (brain degeneration) and Parkinson's (nervous disorder) are very bothersome conditions that prevent a normal life-style.

Consume healthy fats and use your brain to solve mathematical problems, puzzles, crosswords, Sudoku, mysteries, etc. Read a lot and engage in intellectual discussions. Consult a doctor if you experience any awkward development in your behavior.

Skin care

A degenerated skin quickly gives away your age. Subdermal fats get reduced and makes the skin saggy. Take care of warts, moles, folds, wrinkles and dryness. Drink lots of water and stay hydrated. Green tea has Catechin, an antioxidant that's well known for its anti-aging and anti-inflammatory effect. It protects your skin against UV radiation, thus helping to prevent the growth of wrinkles, moles and age spots. You can apply it topically and still get the same anti-aging benefits. Research states that eating four tomatoes a day helps maintain a youthful and disease free skin. Avoid scorching Sun of UV radiation. Moisturizer and sun-screen lotions are good. Collagen supplements, fish oil, coconut oil are good to consume. Pamper your skin and keep the pores clean.

Digestive system

The digestive system slows down because of decreased metabolism with ageing. Drinking enough water and moderate exercise are important things to keep things moving. I advise use of fiber supplements. Eat fiber-rich foods like salads, legumes, unrefined flour and whole fruits instead of pressed juices. Eat small portions, eat less, eat right and mindfully. Eat when hungry. The body performs better when food is digested and stomach is empty. Learn to distinguish between empty, restful stomach and hunger.

No Googling symptoms—No self-medication

The worst thing you can do to yourself is to try becoming a doctor to yourself. Google, or any other search engine, has plenty of data and most of them are un-verified data. For every question there would be volumes of contradictory answers. You will get blown away if you research about symptoms. Try this. Search for cures for the common cold. As you will begin with curcumin and ginger, you will keep on deep diving into causes and cures and common cold will link you up to cancer and scare you terribly.

Similarly, please do not pop up pills just because they are handy. There is no point in following someone else's prescription just because you have similar symptoms.

The year 2020 has witnessed a global pandemic which has exposed several myths about diseases and healthcare. The bottom line lesson was that one has to work on one's immunity and fitness to stay healthy.

Healthcare Insurance

Please afford yourself a healthcare insurance package to the maximum extent of premium you can afford. Cost of medical treatment is becoming beyond the reach of average person hence it would be wise to buy adequate Medi-claim insurance.

Food & Nutrition

1. **Eat Less**: At the foremost, I caution you to eat less and eat wisely. Always eat only up to 80% of your capacity to eat. You need that space in your system to help digest your food. It is likely that you won't get thrilled to hear this, however ongoing experiments found that decreasing calorie consumption remarkably affects the danger of creating illnesses and conditions related with old age — including diabetes, clogged arteries, coronary episodes and strokes

— and can likewise draw out your life! The investigation at Washington University School of Medicine in St. Louis put 25 volunteers aged 41 to 65 on a daily intake of somewhere between 1400 and 2000 calories for over six years. Heart function, circulatory strain and inflammation markers got compared against 25 control subjects, who had a calorie intake of between 2000 to 3000 calories — which is an average of the typical Western diet routine. Heart muscle versatility, pulse and inflammatory markers (counting malignancy related ones) were all essentially more helpful in the low-calorie group. Don't figure you can pull off a supper substitution drink, as the eating regimen, however low in calories, was exceptionally nutritious — rich in olive oil, vegetables, whole grains, fish and natural products.

2. **Consume Anti-oxidants**: As we age, levels of unsafe free radical levels rise, while the body's creation of cell reinforcements, the compounds which can 'mop up' free radicals. As shown by studies at the Human Nutrition Research Center on Aging at Tufts University in Boston, anti-oxidant rich nourishments may slow ageing process in the body and cerebrum. Analysts found that nourishments, for example, blueberries and spinach could expand the anti-oxidant intensity of human blood by 10 to 25 percent.

The cancer prevention nutrients in vitamins A, C and E assume a significant part in securing the body against free radicals, so aim to get your five-a-day, yet in addition ensure that you take in a wide assortment of leafy foods, particularly those of dark colored. Vitamin A specifically assists with keeping the skin healthy, which we get in our eating regimen from nourishments rich in beta-carotene. Carrots are the conspicuous decision — yet yam, pumpkin and melon are likewise acceptable sources.

Vitamin D helped in the counteraction of malignancy in a few experiments and an enormous factor and an enemy of ageing. It is additionally crucial to the combination of collagen which keeps your skin energetic in appearance, and neurotransmitters which keep your brain working in a youthful way. Strangely, many people don't know that Vitamin C likewise has a standard function as an antihistamine to battle that annoying hypersensitivity season. Insufficient vitamin B12 can cause critical and irreparable damage to your nervous system.

Research by Rush University in Chicago in 2005 found that eating oily fish can slow the mental decline associated with aging. The results showed that eating oily fish like salmon at least once a week can slow the rate of cognitive decline by 10 to 13 percent per year.

3. **Eat local, eat natural**: It's pretty common to realize that products of the soil are beneficial for you, particularly when they're in season. Regarding anti-ageing, they are essential. Research proposes that they are the major part of a diet regimen in assisting with preventing age-related sickness. Far better? Eating them promotes a longer life and can forestall the beginning of cognitive issues.

4. **Cut out junk food**: It's pretty common to tie eating an excess of junk food to weight gain and obesity. However, what may come as an astonishment is that eating those low-quality nourishments can likewise negatively affect your emotional well-being and get connected to the annihilation of brain cells. So it is wise to look for signs you're eating such many carbs.

5. **Indulge in moderation**: Eating at a fine-dine restaurant or having a sweet desert are guilty pleasures that many individuals enjoy. However, if you indulge with some restraint, it's OK. Drinking red wine periodically is okay as well, as shown by a research published in Molecules. Also, it may even be beneficial for you. The research suggests that the antioxidants found in red wine can lead to living a longer and healthier life. Resveratrol is a plant compound that acts like an antioxidant. The top food sources include red wine, grapes, some berries and peanuts. This compound mostly

concentrates under the skins and seeds of grapes and berries. However, to get the required dose of resveratrol from red wine, you have to drink a bucketful. Hence these nutrients are best sought through supplements.

Moderate Exercise

Diminishing muscle mass is common with age, especially for men above 30 who may lose as much as 3% to 5% per decade. That loss of muscular mass can contribute to several things, including an increased risk of falls and fractures. Building muscle through lifting weights at home or working out at the gym can help, along with adding extra protein to your diet.

Yoga and Pranayam (regulated breathing) are wonderful habits to develop in anyone's life. Yoga and pranayama are immensely beneficial for the body and mind. Here are some anti-aging yoga postures and pranayama that you can do regularly.

Simhasana (Lion pose) - It reduces tension on the face and chest area. Excellent for enhancing the functioning of a sluggish thyroid gland. Stimulates the platysma (a flat thin muscle in front of the throat) and helps maintain its firmness during the aging process. Helps to remove wrinkles and delays aging. Sit in vajrasana or kneel and keep your knees apart. Keep your palm on the ground in front of you and

bend forward. Keep your eyes open. Now, open your mouth, draw the tongue out and breathe deeply. While breathing, make 'haah!' sound or roar with your tongue outside. Keep the muscles of your stomach, chest and back engaged. Return to the original position and relax.

Vrikshasana (Tree posture) - Vrikshasana strengthens glutes, feet and abs and improves balance. Stand straight with your feet together and arms on the side. Bring your hands to the prayer position and place your left foot on the inner side of the right thigh. Now, inhale and raise your arms above your head. Hold this position for 15 seconds and then come back to the original position. Repeat this asana with your other leg.

Hastpadasana (Standing forward bend) - Prevents inflexibility of the spine that comes with old age. Energizes the nervous system. Hastapadasana will stretch your body and warm up your muscles and joints. Stand straight with your feet together. Keep your knees slightly bent, arms by your side and your toes, forward. Now, inhale and raise your arms slowly above your head. Exhale and bend forward. Make sure that you are bending from your hips. Let your extended arms touch the ground. Hold this position for 10 seconds and return to the original position. Do this asana five times.

Veerbhadrasana (Warrior pose) - Will tone your glutes, calves and knees. Stand straight with feet wide apart. Keep your right foot pointing inward and left foot, outward. Bend your left knee and stretch out your arm. Look at your left arm. Hold this position for ten second and come back to the original position. Now repeat this on the right side. Do this asana five times for each side.

Adho mukha svanasana (Downward facing dog pose) - Improves circulation. Improves digestion, which often gets affected while aging. Tones limbs which get flabby while aging. Decreases anxiety. Adho Mukha Svanasana is an important part of the Suryanamaskara and it improves blood circulation, flexibility and strengthens the spine. Stand straight with your feet apart. Now bend forward and keep your hands on the floor. Your body will form an inverted "V". Keep your core engaged and head hanging. Hold this position for 10 seconds and return to the original position. Repeat this 5 times.

Dhanurasana (Bow pose) - Tones arms and legs muscles which get flabby with age. Energizes the body by stimulating the sympathetic nervous system. Strengthens and relaxes the spine. Start by lying on your stomach on the floor. Inhale and slowly bend your legs backwards. Now, stretch your arms backward and hold on to your ankle. The weight of your body gets supported by your stomach. Hold this position for about 20 seconds and then return to the original position. Repeat this four to five times.

Kapalbhati pranayama (breathing technique) - Removes stress from the eyes and eliminates dark circles. Rejuvenates the brain and energizes the nerves. Calms and uplifts the mind and improves memory. Improves the flow of prana (vital energy) in the body. Gives radiance to the face.

Bharadwajasana (Seated twist) - This asana will tone your abs, reduce double chin and improve flexibility. Sit on the ground with your legs crossed. Keep your left hand on your right knee and your right hand behind you on the floor. Now twist your body and look back. Hold this position for 10 seconds and then return to the original position. Repeat this on the other side.

Take a walk

Going for a stroll outside can transform you — in a genuine sense. An investigation by the University of Michigan found that individuals who went on group nature walks had essentially less depression, lesser stress, and a superior feeling of prosperity. Going outside in the Sun likewise supports vitamin D levels and concentration. Getting that outside air can be as simple as a short walk or hiking a beginner trail in a National Park.

Eat, Sleep, Pray, Repeat

Adopt healthy practices while you are still young Proper sleep cycle, eating right, mindfulness, yoga, regulated breathing, walking etc. are essentials. These practices will slow down the ageing process of your body and mind and keep you healthy by prolonging the biological youth of your body. These will make your biological age much younger than your chronological age and will help you live a healthier life as you grow older. It takes a great deal of time and efforts to develop healthy habits. Some self-help authors claim that it takes 21 days to form a habit, and we can give up good habits with a snap. Another set of authors state that it takes 66 days or more to form a good habit. The crux of the matter is that every person needs some time to develop a new habit. One doesn't start easily with good practices after 60. They have to get inculcated right from the childhood so that your body is agile and your mind is active even as you grow older. With good living habits imbibed in your lifestyle, you are better equipped with a healthy body and mind to live through the old age sans the pains of frailty and disgust.

In this chapter we have learned about how to take care of our physical health. This is the only home of our mind and spirit. In the next chapter we shall delve upon our mental happiness because physical and mental health are the two basic complementing components of a good life.

Key takeaways:

1. We can regulate biological ageing of the body with proper diet, supplements and exercise.

2. Work on your immunity to reduce vulnerability to diseases.

3. Pre-emptive health checks can prevent onset of diseases; and avoid self-medication.

Chapter 2: BE A HAPPY SOUL

"The secret of health for both mind and body is not to mourn for the past, not to worry about the future, or not to anticipate troubles, but to live the present moment wisely and earnestly."—Siddartha Gautama Buddha [Tathagata]

Relationships & family

Studies have announced that the rate of extreme depression among grown-ups aged 65 and above is of somewhere between 2% and 16%, while at anyone point of time to 32% of people aged over 55 feel desolate.

One study found that a large part of nursing home inhabitants without cognitive impedance felt desolate. Like depression, social isolation among older people is significant, with rising patterns among people across the world.

I keep game boards like Monopoly, Life, Scotland Yard, Carrom, Ludo, Snakes & Ladders, a pack of cards and several more things at home and at every given opportunity we share a 'family time' wherein we play, laugh, make noise and enjoy a whale of fun time together.

Spending time together as a family is really one of the most paramount and significant ways we can invest into our kids while they actually live at home.

A sensation of family support is the most valuable blessing we can provide for our kids, making them want to return to that place as grown-ups.

Surrounding ourselves consistently with the individuals who offer love, regard, and positive applause for each other is an astonishing method to bond and shape a hover of trust.

Recall that every individual in your family in a person where they have their own novel contemplations and voices. Permit each other to communicate thoughts of how to develop time all together and afterward grasp those plans to consider approaches to actualize.

Your family is your #1 emotionally supportive network, and are also the individuals who are there with you when you are managing and handling through, disappointments. Control the desire to give those disappointments and feelings to other relatives. They are your support system and the ones who are there to develop you, yet in addition, help you when you fall. Be thoughtful to them. Thoughtfulness starts in your heart and in your home.

Building a home based on trust is significant. We live in a flawed world, encircled by imperfect individuals. Endeavor to make a home to grasp those imperfections while as yet giving encouragement and solutions.

Work on saying 'sorry' and forgiving. We weren't strolling around with awful feelings of resentment because as a family we were learning to apologize, however, to make it right; which made it much simpler for everybody to learn absolution.

East vs West—A contrast of philosophies

In the west there is a feeling of oneself as an element of the Divine wherein life is a service (to the God, money, business, etc.). There is a Linear view of the universe and life, based on the Abrahamic philosophy where everything has its beginning and the end.

In the east, Life is a journey towards eternal realities that are beyond the realities that surround us. There is a circular view of the universe, based on the perception of eternal recurrence.

In the west, there is an emphasis on maximizing happiness because they consider it "ultimate value". We measure happiness in terms of personal achievement and self-fulfillment and focused on achievement of success of the individual.

In the east, happiness is in collectivism. They are more likely to put family or group success over personal success. There is more emphasis on positive relationships and social harmony. They are more likely to resonate with the feelings of others than celebrate their own.

In the west you would search outside yourself - through research and analysis.

In the east you would search inside yourself—by becoming a part of the universe through meditation and holistic living.

In the west your future is unknown, God predetermined it and is not much influenced by your deeds.

In the east, the past and your deeds (karma) today, determine your future.

You might agree or disagree with my philosophy based on the type of conditioning that you have received since your childhood. My philosophies are more inclined to the eastern philosophies because I am conditioned that way.

Happiness should not depend upon the occurrence of some event or achievement of success. It has to be your inner state of mind. *"A joyful person is more likely to be successful whereas a successful person is not necessarily happy."*

You shall be a happier person if you master the art of self-contentment and inner bliss rather than seeking happiness outside from other persons, or events, or material possessions.

I have written a bestseller named "The Secrets to a Magical Life". In this book I have dealt with in detail about how to live a life of fulfillment, purposefulness, and filled with happiness. In this I have explained how life is a flowing stream of time and how you can pick up the jewels of happiness. Those who have read that book before reading this one, might nod in agreement and if not yet read it, then you can explore a large part of my mind through that book.

Keep your friends

"How many slams in an old screen door? Depends how loud you shut it. How many slices in a bread loaf? Depends how thin you cut it. How much good inside a day? Depends how good you live 'em. How much love inside a friend? Depends how much you give 'em."-Shel Silverstein [Author, Cartoonist]

The family that you have just occurred in your life with little choice given to you. To a certain extent one can choose one's spouse, but no other relative comes around at your asking. A friend however is choice that you made at a point of time, because you found him/her as weird as yourself or you simply found a zone of comfort. Keep them forever and pray that they live longer than you. That way you won't have to miss them one by one after attending their funeral and instead they would attend yours and probably share a last laugh remembering how weird you have been.

In a study at Michigan State University, researchers led by William Chopik (Assistant Professor of

Psychology) they reviewed two surveys of approximately 280,000 people. They questioned them about relationships, happiness and health. Chopik said: "As we age, we prune away at some of the friendships that are more superficial and acquaintance-like" and are left "with the ones that are deeper and make us happy." The study reports that older participants identified only by their friendships as reliably powerful predictors of how happy and healthy they felt.

Many studies have shown the positive benefits of friendship on social, emotional and physical well-being. Having a powerful circle of friends can be a good boost for aging hearts and can help the body's autoimmune system resist disease. People who have one or more good friends are in better health than those who have only casual friends or no friends.

Friendship is very important for older people, because of physical changes, loss and retirement. Many people turn to their friends first when they encounter crisis because of the distance of their family. Most times, friends are as important as families.

Studies have found socializing can strengthen the immune system. Socializing can also improve our odds of living longer. Just as loneliness can hurt our health, friendships can actually improve it in far-reaching and surprising ways. It can help us recover more quickly from illness, lower blood pressure and the risk of heart disease, sharpen memory and help us even get a better night's sleep. According to one study, people with powerful connections to family and friends have a 50% greater chance of outliving those with fewer social ties.

Your friend or friend group can serve as a support system for you, especially if they are around the same age as you. If you are dealing with the loss of a loved one or with limited mobility, your group of friends likely is experiencing the same thing or something similar. They can give you advice that your junior family members simply cannot give you, because of lack of experience or understanding. Your friends will serve as your support system during a time of change that many people call lonely and scary.

Live your own life

Old age is an incredible chance to kick back and make the most of your life. You are a lot wiser, so opinions of others ought not fluster you. You are considerably more at ease with yourself. Your children may have ventured out from home, and you do all the things you need to do.

Studies revealed, happy seniors experienced less difficulty getting up, dressing, or cleaning up, instead of unhappy seniors who were twice as prone to the risk of diabetes, coronary illness, malignancy, and strokes.

Research has shown that a strong sense of direction for seniors had a defensive impact. Individuals who kept in contact with loved ones remained sound in their old age. An examination on centenarians showed they clutched an unequivocal reason in their lives through dealing with grandkids, incredible grandkids, and chipping in.

Continue refreshing yourself with the most recent on news, innovation, music, books, films. Keep a pleasant sense of dressing dapper and do not become a minimalist too soon after retirement. It sounds cool initially to give up on things you have been doing all your life and adopt the staple basics, but after sometime you will get bored with yourself and to people around you.

Stay active, go out for walks, join a club to play cards, or a volunteer care group. Interact with people every day. I know an old man who could barely walk, but he made it his routine to strut along slowly in the nearby park where small children of the poor folks would wait for him because he goes there and teaches them how to read and write in an open classroom.

Making yourself outdated is the worst thing you can do to yourself. Beware of the Rip Van Winkle syndrome. Do not get entangled in the time warps and never say that in your times things were like that and it is not the same nowadays. Become a part of the transformation. Keep accepting and mastering the changes in technology and society. Let this be your own era as long as you live.

While your children are kids, do not take decisions on their behalf. Help them learn how to take decisions instead. This way you will make them more independent, matured and wiser, and they will not need you to solve their problems for a lifetime. That means lesser stress for you in your golden years. If they still come to seek your advice, then share your point of view through your experience and knowledge, without totally empathizing and still leave it to them to decide.

Practice your hobby

"Try new hobbies. Develop new interests. Pursue new experiences. When you expand your interests, you increase your opportunities for happiness."
— Richelle E. Goodrich [Author]

For seniors, intellectually testing exercises are significant. They help to keep the mind working at a significant level. Creative art is a pleasant method to remain intellectually dynamic. It offers genuine intellectual advantages. As shown by an article from Today's Geriatric Medicine, the most recent neurological research shows that craftsmanship delivers new neural pathways and reinforces dendrites. It implies that there is convincing proof that craftsmanship helps to enhance brain function. Hobbies contribute to significant benefits such as self-articulation. Creative art is really a psychological exercise. It can assist with keeping an individual's brain working appropriately profoundly into their later years.

Individuals above 65 spend a normal of 10 hours daily either sitting or lying down, making them the most inactive age group. Keeping in mind that growing health constraints can limit one's capacity to get out and do specific kinds of activity, there are still diversions that you can appreciate that can help you remain dynamic.

The National Institute on Aging reports that there are many advantages that seniors can pick up by giving some an ideal opportunity for doing an activity or taking part in a hobby. Some of these advantages include:

- A diminished danger for creating medical conditions, for example, dementia.

- A longer life expectancy.

- An increased rate of feeling upbeat and sound.

- A more noteworthy ability to be self-efficacy.

- Increased flexibility even with misfortune and stress.

- Improved memory, cognizance, innovativeness, and critical thinking aptitudes

Contingent upon your inclinations, there are a great deal of choices seniors have, when searching for an interest or hobby to appreciate.

There is a tremendous amount of emotional well-being if you care for your pet. It gives a sense of belongingness and companionship beside security.

Gardening is a healthy activity that provides a physical work-out and mental satisfaction at the same time.

I knew an elder who played violin and could happily be with himself for hours with no worries bothering him at all.

Deal with your anxiety & depression

"Every man has his secret sorrows which the world knows not; and often times we call a man cold when he is only sad." −Henry Wadsworth Longfellow [Poet & Educator]

Depression is something other than feeling miserable or blue. It is a typical yet genuine temperament problem that needs treatment. It causes serious manifestations that influence how you feel, think, and handle day to day routine, for example, sleeping, eating, and working.

At the point when you have depression, you experience difficulty with day-to-day life for quite a long time at a time. Specialists call this condition "depressive disorder" or "clinical depression."

Depression is a genuine sickness. It's anything but a sign of an individual's shortcoming or a character blemish. You can't "wake up from" clinical depression. The vast majority who experience depression need treatment to improve.

For example, the demise of a friend or family member, retirement from work, or managing a genuine ailment can leave individuals feeling tragic or restless. After a time of change, many grown-ups can recover their passionate equilibrium, yet others don't and may develop depression.

There are a few sorts of depressive issues.

Significant grief includes extreme side effects that meddle with the capacity to work, rest, study, eat, and appreciate life. An episode can happen just a single time in an individual's lifetime, however more regularly, an individual has a few episodes.

Persistent depressive disorder is a depressed state of mind that goes on for 2 or more years. An individual diagnosed with persistent depressive disorder may have episodes of significant depression alongside times of less serious side effects, yet manifestations should keep going for a very long time to get viewed as constant depressive disorder.

Different types of depression include psychotic depression, post birth anxiety, and occasional seasonal disorder.

There are many indications related with depression, and some will shift contingent upon the person. They recorded the absolute most basic side effects beneath. On the off chance that you have a few of these side effects for over about fourteen days, you may have depression.

- Persistent dismal, on edge, or "void" disposition
- Feelings of sadness, blame, uselessness, or weakness
- Irritability, fretfulness, or experiencing difficulty sitting still
- Loss of interest in once pleasurable exercises, including sex
- Decreased energy or weakness
- Moving or talking all the more slowly
- Difficulty concentrating, recollecting and deciding
- Difficulty in sleeping, waking up early, or over sleeping
- Eating pretty much than expected, normally with impromptu weight gain or misfortune
- Thoughts of death or self-destruction, or attempts of self-destruction
- Aches or torments, cerebral pains, spasms, or stomach related issues without an unmistakable actual reason and that don't ease with treatment
- Frequent crying

Gloom, even a serious one, can get dealt with. On the off chance that you figure you may have depression, start by planning to see your primary care physician or medical services supplier. This could be your essential specialist or a medico who works in diagnosing and treating psychological wellness conditions (a psychologist or psychiatrist). Certain drugs and some ailments can cause similar indications as despondency. A specialist can prevent these conceivable outcomes by doing an actual test, meeting, and lab tests. If the specialist can locate no ailment that might cause the downturn, the subsequent stage is a mental assessment.

Consider talking with your doctor about sensitive subjects, including depression and mental health.

Treatment decisions vary for every individual, and we should attempt sometimes different medicines to discover the one that works. It is essential to continue attempting until you discover something that works for you.

The most widely recognized types of treatment for depression are medicine and psychotherapy.

How to prevent onset of depression?

1. Get informed—Know what is right and read only from the right sources. So much of fake news on the pandemic 2019-20 went around through various media that terrified people.

Restrict your newsfeed. Get the right information before you panic.

2. Social contacts are important. Stay in touch with distant folks in the family through social media and also join a local social activity group or join your friends for a bonhomie. Try to help others and be useful so you can bask in the glory of good deeds.

3. Limit the use of substances, smoking, drinking, and other intoxicants. They worsen the situation.

4. Follow a daily routine:
   - Wake up and go to sleep at similar times every day to maintain your circadian rhythm.
   - Exercise regularly—whatever your body is used to, whether yoga, walking, or light exercise.
   - Allocate time for working and time for resting.
   - Keep up with personal hygiene. Besides the body, tidy up your surroundings as well.
   - Eat healthy meals at regular time intervals and also take care of your supplements.
   - Make time for doing things you enjoy.
   - Meditate—ideally you should meditate for 30 minutes each in the morning and evening. Meditation keeps you calm and

focused and connects you well with your inner self.

How to Meditate?

One can do 'Mindful' meditation, anywhere, anytime. Sit in a quiet and comfortable place in a calm posture, close your eyes and focus your attention inward to a fixed point between your eyes. You are mindful of the world around you, but without reacting. Focus on your controlled breathing. Inhale slowly at the count of 1-2-3, to fill your lungs to full capacity, and then hold your breath 1-2, and then exhale at the count of 1-2-3-4. This is the ideal rhythm of breathing that one must practice all the time. Like Zen master Thich Nhat Hanh says: *"Feelings come and go like clouds in a windy sky. Conscious breathing is my anchor."* This is an excellent relaxation technique wherein one is restful but not asleep.

Another method is 'transcendental' meditation wherein you play some favorite mantra or natural sounds or tunes to help focus and concentrate with lesser effort than a mindful meditation and follow the same as that.

Guided meditation is in the care of a Guru or teacher who speaks in a manner to give you an imagery to focus upon. It is like Neuro Linguistic

Programming, where voice commands are used for the imagery.

There is also meditation, along with certain postures of yoga that require greater balance. Maintaining the balance of postures helps to focus and concentrate better with no distraction. It requires more practiced effort for the Chakra meditation or awakening the 'Kundali'. It is a calm posture like the mindful meditation but it gets done preferably in early morning hours after complete fasting through the night. It is a reverberation method wherein you focus on the path of your spine beginning from the anus and travel up step by step through belly, chest, throat, forehead and the top of the head. Chanting "AUM" in a base tone helps to reverberate and awaken the chakras hidden in your organs. It will require a lot of practice and the day you touch upon the fontanel you will experience bliss. The art of meditation is over-rated as an exclusive expertise, but it is much simpler.

Meditation must be a part of our daily routine. Though any time of the day when it is possible for you, it should be fine if that works for you, but early hours of the morning are the best ones.

Meditation helps to reduce stress. In fact, this is the key takeaway. It helps to control anxiety and promotes emotional health. It helps to enhance self-awareness and also helps to expand your attention span. Meditation also helps in improving memory and stops the degeneration of brain cells because of ageing. It is a major enabler for mental, emotional and spiritual well-being. The mystical Osho said: *"Touch your inner space, which is nothingness, as silent and empty as the sky; it is your inner sky. Once you settle down in your inner sky, you have come home, and great maturity arises in your actions, in your behavior. Then whatever you do has grace in it. Then whatever you do is a poetry in itself. You live poetry; your walking becomes dancing, your silence becomes music."*

[How to meditate is adapted from "The Secrets to a Magical Life"]

In this chapter we have learned about the importance of family, friends and peers in life because humans are social animals. Practicing hobbies helps one engage with self. Anxiety and depression are inevitable, but we can deal with them. We have also learned how to meditate and connect with the universe.

In the next chapter we shall learn about how one can stay active & agile to live a purposeful life. We shall also learn from live examples how to play the second innings in life after retiring from the first.

> *Key takeaways:*
>
> 1. *Keep your kin and friends close because they can help you share your happiness.*
>
> 2. *We cannot avoid but can deal with anxiety and depression.*
>
> 3. *Practicing hobbies and meditation are few best ways to connect with self and the universe.*

Chapter 3: STAY ACTIVE & AGILE

"If you feel rooted in your home and family, if you're active in your community, there's nothing more empowering. The best way to make a difference in the world is to start by making a difference in your own life."-Julia Louis-Dreyfus [actress, comedian, singer and producer]

Do not sit idle or become home-bound

It is okay to watch television for sake of news, information or entertainment, as long as you have allocated yourself a specific time slot for doing that. Imagine if you have to do it all day long just to pass your time away, then I would call it a torture.

Broadly, there are 3 types of activities you can engage into:

1. Gainful work

2. Recreation

3. Social work

Gainful Work

Do you believe that age is just a number? There is a minimal difference in the work performance potential of a 60 years old compared to someone at 40. It does not limit physical endurance to age, but it is all about how well you follow a fitness regime. However, those in a salaried job have to retire after attaining a certain age because of regulations and policies and not because he/she has become worthless. One who is used to working 8 to 10 hours a day at the workplace feels a sudden void after retirement, and this is one of the major reasons for feeling melancholy. It pinches more when money stops flowing into your bank account. Those in business usually have a longer stint at work till the time they find some dependable young hand to transfer their responsibilities to. Hence it is imperative for everyone to think at their young age about how they are going to shape up a roadmap for the future. It is difficult to start new things after 60. Although age isn't a limitation either. While Barack Obama retired at 55, Donald Trump took over the White House at 74. Then you have a Joe Biden who, at 78, gears up to take over the oval office. His wife and daughter died in an accident while going to purchase a Christmas tree. His son died because of cancer. Another son removed from U.S. Navy because of substance abuse. He himself had face muscles in paralysis. He never gave up.

Here are some interesting stories from Rohan Paul about late bloomers to inspire you.

Mc Donalds

Beam Kroc was 52 years of age in 1954. He was a milkshake machine sales rep. One day he occurred on a hamburger stand in San Bernardino, California, and instead of selling the McDonald siblings his machine, he purchased their business. Following 6 years, by 1960, Kroc had over 200

McDonald establishments in the U.S. Kroc said: *"Luck is the dividend of sweat. The more you sweat, the luckier you get."*

Honda

In the 1940s, Soichiro Honda made a motorbike by connecting a little motor to a bicycle. This achievement drove him to planning a small bike. He was 42 years of age when he launched the Honda Motor Company in 1948, and within 10 years of beginning Honda, he was the main bike producer on the planet. By 1988, at 82 years, he and his organization already entered world's Automobile Hall of Fame. Honda said, *"Success represents the 1% of your work, which results from the 99% that is called failure."*

J. K. Rowling

By 1993, 28 years old J. K. Rowling, after a fleeting marriage, a miscarriage, and afterward turning into a single parent, she was a failure by common norms. She was jobless, separated, destitute, and with a dependent kid. She endured episodes of melancholy in the long run, pursuing government-aided help. At that base most point, to cite her own words — she pondered internally, "I actually had an old typewriter and a major thought". In 1995, Rowling completed her composition for "Harry

Potter and the Philosopher's Stone" however, each of the 12 significant distributers dismissed the Harry Potter content. A year later, a small distributing house, Bloomsbury, acknowledged it and advanced her a little £1500 advance. In 1997, when she was 32, the book was distributed with just 1000 copies, 500 of which got circulated to libraries. The rest is history. Rowling said: *"Rock bottom became the solid foundation on which I rebuilt my life."*

KFC

Harland David Sanders was a series of disappointments who got terminated from dozen jobs. Begging the proprietors of run-down burger joints to use his recipe and give him a nickel commission on every chicken. He slept in the rear of his car and made handshake bargains. He opened a restaurant to sell his special chicken. At age 65, his own eatery was bankrupt. Presently resigned from his positions, he liquidated his first Social Security check and Kentucky Fried Chicken (KFC) got conceived. He was so sure about his capacity to pressure fry the chicken that he used the last cash he had and put it in his café. 10 years later, Sanders had over 600 Kentucky Fried Chicken establishments in the U.S. and in Canada as well. Sanders said: *"I made a resolve then, that I was going to amount to something."*

Grandma Moses

Anna Mary Robertson Moses was initially a major fanatic of embroidery, however once her arthritis became excessively agonizing for her to hold a needle, she checked painting out during the 1930s. She was 76 when she turned out her first canvas, and she lived another 25 years as a painter. Her works have appeared and got sold in the United States and abroad and have got showcased on greetings cards and other product. Moses' works of art are among the collections of many historical centers. 'The Sugaring Off' got sold for US$1.2 million out of 2006.

Julia Child

Julia Child was 49 years of age when her first cookbook, Mastering the Art of French Cooking, got distributed. At 51 years of age she picked up TV fame cooking show, which debuted in 1963. At 69 years old, she became co-founder of the American Institute of Wine and Food to help promote the information on food and wine through eateries. In 1984, at 72 years old, she finished a series of 6 videotapes about "The Way to Cook". Before the end of 1965, The French Chef was conveyed by 96 PBS stations. Sales of "Mastering the Art of French Cooking" were picking up — 200,000 copies sold. In 1966, she won an Emmy. Time put her on the cover in a feature article on American food — "Everybody's in the Kitchen." As of late, they made Hollywood movies based on her life. Julia said: *"The measure of achievement is not winning awards. It is doing something that you appreciate, something you believe is worthwhile."*

These are just a few pearls from the ocean of high achievers who never allowed their age to come into their way. They followed their inner calling at whatever age they could and made a humble beginning. They all had in them two things.

1. Persistence; 2. Perseverance

Persistence is a firm or obstinate continuance in a course of action despite difficulty or opposition; perseverance is the steadfastness in doing something despite difficulty or delay in achieving success. It is the art of not giving up.

At a point of time, most of us picked up a job or a career because that's what came by our way. You can stay active even if you are trading on the stock exchange, or you give online lectures, or you become an author and/or mentor, or and editor or a designer. Just identify your talent, bring it out and put it to use. Every person has some hidden persona inside him/her that needs to come out.

Follow your calling irrespective of your age. Your mission on this planet is unfulfilled until you have given to the world what is due from you. Indian author Deepak Chopra said: *"In every seed is the promise of thousands of forests, but the seed must not be hoarded; it must give its intelligence to the fertile ground. Through its giving, its unseen energy flows into material manifestation."* So do not stop your energy. Keep it flowing in circulation lest it might stagnate and solidify much like the blood which stays liquid while it flows and solidifies into a clot once it stops flowing.

Recreation

The reason I did not say 'recreation work', is because recreation is no work. Stay active enough in life to do all your chores by yourself. Having allocated enough time for whatever you have to do indoors, including resting, you ought to have an outdoorsy plan as well. It is imperative to go out and get some Sun. Going for a walk or walking your pet should be a definite thing on your agenda. Besides, engage into some recreational games. Even visiting temples is a good idea. They do a lot of chanting there, which can support you to engage into transcendental meditation.

The important part here is that your recreational activities must have two aspects.

1. We should do it every day

2. There has to be a time slot allocated for this

If you keep it optional, you would end up never doing them. It takes about three weeks to build a habit, but a habit can get destroyed much sooner than that. Do not give it away to change of weather or minor health issues. Re-schedule your plans and find means to work around the situations. Regularity in recreation also helps you to develop an attitude for being regular at work.

"All work and no play makes Jack's grandparent a dull person."

Social work

Many of you are blessed with financial stability in life. Apparently you do not need to work for earning some income through your activities. That makes you an ideal choice for contributing your time and efforts towards social work. Anybody can donate money towards charity but what it requires of you is your time, efforts and experienced advice.

Become a part of a social help group. You can do a lot by yourself alone. You can give tuitions to poor children at a park under the tree, you could go around representing peoples' cause, you could provide healthcare, but when you do that all alone, there are greater chances of your efforts and energy fizzing out some day. When you join a social group or form one with like-minded seniors, then you build a greater synergy. You can pool in resources and organize things in a better way. When you go alone, you could go faster, but when you go together, you can go further.

Politics is not a dirty word at all. It is a work which requires high involvement with people. This rubs in a lot of power because you represent the people who stand behind you. It is up to you how you use this power. You can use it constructively for general welfare or you can abuse it for personal selfish gains. Eventually it is your own character that determines whether an activity is good. You must have also noticed with astonishment that politicians often live an endless life as compared to others because they get constantly charged up with their engagement with people. As soon as they quit from active public life, they perish soon. Thus, if you involve yourself in some work which gives you the opportunity to interact with people, then it helps you live healthier and longer.

Winston Churchill should be the best light of hope to every politician. He failed secondary school multiple times. He went through his whole grown-up time on earth as a political disappointment, losing each offer for public office ... until he at last became the prime minister of England at the mature age of 62. Churchill said: *"You've got enemies? Good. That means you've stood up for something, sometime in your life."*

A. C. Bhaktivedanta Swami Prabhupada - the originator of ISKCON, or the 'Hare Krishna' movement, was 69 years of age before he founded the International Society for Krishna Consciousness (ISKCON).

In his native India, Prabhupada had been a chemist and a Sanskrit researcher in Kolkata (erstwhile Calcutta), yet in 1965, at 69, he came to New York City with only fifty bucks, a pair of cymbals, and a longing to spread the teachings of Lord Krishna. His journey was not supported by any religious association, nor got welcomed upon his arrival by a gathering of faithful devotees.

Prabhupada got off to a humble beginning by sitting on a walkway in the East Village and chanting. However, by the time he passed away in 1977 he emerged as a significant figure of the Western non-conformity, starting a movement with many youthful Americans.

In the twelve years from his appearance in New York until his last days, he traveled around the world 14 times on lecture tours, initiated thousands of supporters, established the religious settlement New Vrindaban in West Virginia, composed over eighty books, watched ISKCON develop to a confederation of over 550 centers, including 60 farm networks, some focusing on self-sufficiency, 50 schools and different activities the world over.

These examples are to explain how age can never be a barrier for anyone who wants to go out and connect with the masses. If you have it in you, then just bring it out to the people.

In this chapter we learned how one can re-launch a fresh career or continue with one for a long time.

One must not stop oneself to seek recreation in life. Also, social work is an engaging method to share your learning with the society. In the next chapter we shall learn how to be financially independent during those golden years to live with more confidence.

<u>*Key takeaways:*</u>

1. *You have the potential to relaunch your fresh career when you are older.*

2. *Seek various means of recreation and live your life zestfully.*

3. *Give back to the society by engaging in social work.*

Part 2: Financial Independence

Chapter 4: BE FINANCIALLY WISE

"You must gain control over your money, or the lack of it will forever control you."–Dave Ramsey [Author cum radio host]

The world has its own callous ways to retire a person from employment and stop his/her income when money is in fact required for a decent living. Some jobs offer a lifelong pension, but most jobs don't. Also, if you are into a profession which is built around you or if you own a small enterprise which is also about just you in the core team, then you are heading for a hard grind in your old age. Anticipate these situations while you are still young and save enough for those days.

At the outset let me introduce you to another of my bestseller book called, "How to Grow Rich & Become Wealthy." In this book, I have explained about how to make a life plan. How to assess how much money we shall require, and at what stage in life? How much to save? How to save? Where to invest? How to take care of your investments? How to create wealth for meeting all future needs at various milestones in life? Reading this book would give you adequate knowledge and confidence about managing your finances, and you shall become financially wise.

During your old age and as long as you live, you will require money for mainly 3 things:

1. For the day-to-day living expenses.

2. For growing cost of medical care.

3. For recreation and fun.

The age for retirement remains fixed, but nobody knows for how many years one shall live after retirement. You will constantly require money for your day-to-day living expenses. The cost of living always increases year on year, and accordingly you ought to have saved into such an annuity that pays you enough every year to cover all your expenses. Do not rely upon eating into your capital funds because you never know, you might outlive your reserves.

The next major need for money is for your growing medical expenses. You will spend more on healthcare as you grow older, so you add some comfort to your deteriorating body. Some countries have social security schemes to take care of those expenses, but several countries don't. If you live in a country that does not support you for this, then you must work upon building a corpus for eldercare expenses as well. Most insurance companies cover your health insurance during your younger days, but stop insuring you after you become old.

It is necessary to have enough money for your recreation and fun as well. You have worked hard all your life, and it is your right to live a comfortable life full of recreation and fun. We cannot undermine the need for this. Imagine if you have no work and no recreation either, then what would remain in life to live for? Hence a budget should get provided for recreation as well.

I write this book for people who are still young so they gain adequate insight into the requirements for their future. You cannot end up at 60 with no corpus of funds and no pension income to sustain. This book is all about the preparedness for a sunshine future during a golden sunset. The sooner you realize this, and work upon it, the stronger you end up as a senior citizen.

Things to do for financial adequacy

1. **Save**—One has to save out of what one earns. Ideally, save 30% of your earning first before you spend. During the period you are earning, follow the equation:

   $$\text{Income} - \text{Savings} = \text{Expenditure}$$

   It implies that you must first achieve your targeted savings before you spend, because if the amount left over after spending were to be your savings, then you could never save enough.

2. **Do not waste**- Consumption and utilization of resources is one thing, and wasting them away is another thing. Follow three principles of consumption:
   (i) Do not buy what you don't need.

(ii) Buy only as much as you can consume.
(c) Do not waste what you have bought.

Money saved is money earned. If you follow these three principles of consumption, you will subtly build enough additional resources. For example, the average U.S. retail price of cigarettes is $6.65 per pack. Americans who smoke one pack a day, therefore, spend about $2427.25 a year. If you compound this monthly over 10 years at an assumed rate of interest @ 5% then you would have spent $31,367. Imagine if you quit smoking and save this money. Likewise, there are other wasteful habits of useless consumption.

3. **Invest wisely**–Your money should earn money for you without needing your presence and hard work. This means you should invest in an asset class which either generates a regular income or can get sold at a profit in a short/long term. If you bought a lavish bungalow or an expensive car, then it is not an investment. You are not earning rent from that bungalow, you cannot sell your home for an appreciated valuation, and the car is anyway a depreciating asset.

Invest in a commercial property that earns rent for you or invest into the stock market. If you find these investments big ticket or volatile, then grow your wealth through investing into mutual funds. They give you a good return in a long run.

How much to invest in a risk bearing volatile asset class vis-à-vis how much to invest in a guaranteed returns investment? You may follow the thumb rule of 100 minus age. Say your age is 60. So 100-60=40. It implies that 40% of your investment portfolio can be into high risk—high returns schemes and the rest into guaranteed returns scheme.

4. **Consolidate**—It will require a lot of time, energy and efforts for conversion into cash, when you need the money, if your assets and investments are scattered and are lying in various forms of assets that require a lot of your time and monitoring. So merge the fragmented assets gradually into a more manageable form of asset class that generates regular income.

5. **Get rid of debt**—Make sure you do not have loans to repay after your retirement. It also implies that you should not leave behind liabilities for your family to suffer with. You cannot justify the interest you pay on your debts unless you have invested the money into an income generating asset. The income that gets generated should offset the interest cost.

6. **Document**—Maintain proper documents of your investments and share its whereabouts with a trusted family member. There could be times when you might need someone to help you with them. It is also wise to maintain wherever possible, a joint ownership with your spouse or nearest kin.

7. **Will**—Make a living will. It is a document of self-declaration wherein you mention clearly about

your list of assets and investments and nominate your benefactor (s) after you. Make sure that your benefactor has the original document of your will, else he/she may not get what you bequeath on him/her. Nobody can claim a better title other than the benefactor who holds the original document of your will.

Manage your financial matters yourself

Learn to manage your financial matters yourself.

You make seek help of a trusted member in your family but you must keep your fingers on the tab.

You should be able to manage your wealth by yourself in your own personal interest.

Do not give away all your wealth during your lifetime. Factor in the darker facets of life.

Convert your high-risk exposure to more of guaranteed returns portfolio.

Learn the technology for online bank operation, tax returns filing, operating and transacting through Demat account, monitoring your transactions online. Develop a full stack brain. Never say no to technology. This will help you keep control and monitoring over your finances.

Do not succumb to cheats and fraudsters, who are on a prowl to fleece your money by exploiting your ignorance.

Laws to safeguard the security of elders

This is not to construe as a legal opinion or advice but stated for sake of worthy information. Be aware of laws of the land that safeguards the elders from being forced into destitution by their own over ambitions children.

Maintenance and Welfare of Parents and Senior Citizens Act, 2007 is a legislation, started by the Ministry of Social Justice and Empowerment, Government of India to provide more effective provision for maintenance and welfare of parents and senior citizens. It makes it a legal obligation for children and heirs to provide maintenance to senior citizens and parents by monthly allowance. It also provides simple, speedy and inexpensive mechanism for protecting life and property of the older persons.

Several states in the U.S. have passed filial (due from a son or daughter) responsibility laws. These filial responsibility laws require the adult children to provide financial support to their parents if they cannot take care of themselves or to cover unpaid medical bills, such as assisted living or long-term care costs. This also includes food, clothing, shelter, and health care/medical needs of the parent.

England's Poor Law of 1601 stated that communities met the needs of the poor elderly, but only after the resources of adult children got exhausted.

China's constitution requires that adult children fulfill their duty to care for aging parents, but the government supplements this aid through public pensions and a state income maintenance program for select elders.

Many countries have tried to articulate who handles the welfare of dependent family members via the creation of laws.

In this chapter we have learned about the various things one requires money for. We have also learned how to save and invest wisely and about other financial prudence. We have understood the importance of managing the money by self. Also, most developed nations have laws to safeguard the financial needs of the elders. In the next chapter we shall learn how to live in a secure environment.

> ### _Key takeaways:_
>
> 1. _Various needs for money and various ways to invest safely._
>
> 2. _Manage your money yourself._
>
> 3. _Know the laws that mandates your kin to take care you in your old age._

Part 3: Safety and Security

Chapter 5: SAFETY AT HOME

"There is nothing more important than a safe and secure home."

Elders staying alone without support from younger kin are vulnerable to certain risks. They need to adopt some precautions to stay safe at home.

Telephone with emergency numbers

Every senior citizen must have access to a telephone and a list of emergency contact numbers. Numbers of nearest kin, emergency contact numbers, neighbors, family doctor, ambulance, police, pharmacy and grocery store must be handy. Better still, some emergency numbers must get updated as hot-keys.

If you are staying far from your aged parents, make sure they have access to call someone in times of emergency.

For the elders, it is always good to have a fixed landline telephone in their living room. Mobile phones can have connectivity issues or the battery might run out our ring-tone might get silenced. They get panicked soon unless there is a steady back-up.

Emergency alarms

Invest in fire alarms and burglar / intruder alarms, preferably with hooter to alarm the neighbors in case any mishap happens.

Program the telephone for a one button sprint call to the local police station, fire station and ambulance.

These alarms will assist to garner faster response in case the senior citizen has slowed down in their response.

It may sound paranoid and over precaution, but these small arrangements can make a big difference in their lives.

Magic eye and surveillance

Old people living alone are vulnerable to daylight robbery by unscrupulous people barging inside their house on some pretext. There are several instances of seniors being attacked at home by intruders.

Install magic eye and safety chains on main doors so that one can safely check before opening the doors accidentally to a stranger.

Young adults staying away from aged parents because of job or other commitments can enable remote surveillance through internet based CCTV cameras installed at home.

Sometimes the attackers are accomplices of their helpers and maids. While appointing a helper, nurse or maid, it is good to have their police verification and background check done through the police or recruiting agency.

Prevent falls on wet floors

Accidental falls in old age can be painful, bone breaking and sometimes fatal.

Use anti-skidding rubber mats in bathrooms and kitchen to avoid fall because of slipping on the wet floor.

Sometimes a moment of dizziness because of any health reasons can become a cause for a fall.

Persons who have difficulty in walking or balancing themselves during walking should better use walker supports.

Highly disabled persons can use motored wheel chairs.

Safety of valuables and documents

Old people may have temporary loss of memory and may forget where important documents and valuables got kept. They need to have just one designated place to keep all valuables and important documents.

We should keep all valuables and documents in a vault. Invest in a vault if you do not have one already.

Commercial banks also offer vaults on rent, but then they are away from home and there has to be some safe vault at home as well.

Variable levels of flooring

For a young person, a contoured flooring seems cool with a step or two going downwards into the living room or a duplex house looks quite compact.

If your house or apartment has variable levels of flooring, then it could become an impediment for the elders.

It is better to have one uniform level of flooring.

Repairs and Maintenance

The house or apartment has to get periodically repaired and well maintained. Loose wiring, leaky pipes, broken window panes and other irregularities can become bothersome and hazardous for the old people at home.

In this chapter we learned about some basic precautions and some special arrangements necessary for the safety of the aged at home. In the next chapter we shall read about the safety precautions outside home.

<u>*Key takeaways:*</u>

1. *Create an environment at home which is safe for the older people.*

2. *Emergency alarms and surveillance systems are essential.*

3. *Check the design element and the maintenance of your home to maintain safety at home.*

Chapter 6: SAFETY OUTSIDE HOME

"Make safety a part of your lifestyle. Keep safety at every step of your life."

Nobody can and should never be home bound. While moving out of home for a regular errand, work, leisure, walk, doctor visit, social work or any other reason, there are concerns about the safety of the elders.

ID card and contact info

When the elders go for a walk or activities outside home, always keep an identification card in your pocket with emergency contact numbers.

Sometimes one can faint because of hypoglycemia or hypertension or a fall injury. The card comes handy to identify the victim, rush them to the hospital and inform his/her kin.

Carry a mobile phone

While out for a walk, carry your mobile phone with you and make sure you have access to important emergency numbers. Who knows, you may need to reach or someone or your family and friends need to reach you.

Prevent falls on pavement and parks

Make sure you have all the things with you to help prevent accidental falls.

It is common to see such accidents happen when someone mindlessly rams into an elder or reckless driving.

Bag snatchers

Old people are vulnerable to get way-laid and attacked. If confronted, do not resist. Never carry too much valuables with you. Do carry a can of pepper spray or an electric stunner to combat a way layer in case of urgency.

Companion along

It is always wise to move out along with a companion. Be that your spouse or grandchild or an attendant.

If there is someone with you, then you are a lot more confident and a helping hand is near you.

Pandemic precaution

The pandemic situation in 2020 has taught many precautions.

Wear a mask, use sanitizer, do not touch things unnecessarily, stay away from crowded places.

In this chapter we learned how to cater to the safety needs of the elders when they are out of home. In the next chapter, we shall read about safety precautions during traveling.

Key takeaways:

1. *Stay safe outside with a little preparedness.*

2. *Prevent injury and robbery.*

3. *Extra precaution during pandemic is a must.*

Chapter 7: TRAVEL SAFE

"Some have eyes and cannot see; Some have ears and cannot hear; So be wise and wear your safety gear."

I always recommend traveling for the aged people. After a dint of hard work all your life, it is time now to travel and see the world beyond your work life. You have all the time and there are things lying in your bucket list to tick off some day. Traveling far from home needs some extra preparation for seniors. There has to be preparedness for your essentials, and also some special measures are required.

Prior Planning

It is wise to make all the bookings upfront for your stay and travel. Prior bookings keep you stress free and well prepared. You get well received when you land up at a place where you got booked in already.

Once a friend advised me to travel without booking a room at a resort. He told me with his over-confidence that you can really strike a last-minute deal if you just land there because the guys at the resort would be desperate to fill in a vacant room. It happened otherwise. They were full already. Then instead of bargaining, I had to request to accommodate me. They obliged me with a shoddy room, which nobody checks in otherwise. I learned a lesson of a lifetime.

If you are not driving by yourself and it is a long drive, then hire a chauffeur or cab from an agency known to you. As a measure of precaution, I do not recommend stranger radio taxis.

GPS Monitoring

Give access of your geo positioning to a responsible kin so they can track you if needed. Also ensure that you know how to use a GPS navigation system to find your way. Every smart phone nowadays has an app to guide the route for anywhere in the world. It is good for everyone how to use it, instead of asking directions from strangers, so you ride with confidence and nobody takes you for a ride.

Avoid posting your plans on social media

Beware if you are posting your holiday plans on social media. You may offer clues to someone to break into your vacant house behind you. No matter how cool it appears, but publishing too much personal content on social media is not a good idea. There are cyber crooks lurking around to follow posts from naïve people to plan a massive house-break in their absence of way lay them on a lonely highway.

Eat safe

Highway motels may seem to be a good place to eat, but eat safely and watch out for the hygiene maintained at those places.

There are some places in the world where they serve bizarre cuisines that are beyond you. Play safe with fruits, bread, and juices in such places.

It is always a good idea to stock up some snacks, fruits and juice cans in the boot of your car, just in case you do not find a reliable place to eat.

Medicines

Keep your medicines, supplements, and prescriptions handy. It is pointless to mention, but people often forget to keep them handy and pack them off down below in their suitcase. They might miss some doses that are essential for life support.

Water

Go for safe packaged water while traveling instead of trying to drink water from taps and any natural sources. It takes time for anyone to get accustomed to water at a different place. There are chances of getting diahorrea because of unclean water. Same with freshly pressed juices. You cannot be sure about the hygiene standards followed, hence packaged ones are more safe to have. I mention these safety concerns not to scare you or cause any panic, but to raise your awareness for the need for preparedness. With changing times, simple things are giving way to complexities.

In this chapter we learned about preparing for a safe travel and about precautions to take during travel. In the next chapter we shall learn about cyber security and how to be safe in this digital world.

Key takeaways:

1. *Make safe travel arrangements prior.*

2. *Do not publish your travel plans / pictures on social media.*

3. *Take care of your food, supplements and medicines during travel.*

Chapter 8: CYBER SECURITY

"Passwords are like underwear: don't let people see it, change it very often, and you shouldn't share it with strangers."—Chris Pirillo [Tech TV host]

We are already into the future and we are living in a cyber-world where internet, online transactions and internet of things (IOT) are inevitable. Here are a few words of caution for everyone, and for the seniors in particular.

1) Train yourself to be tech savvy—As long as you live, this world belongs to you and the technological developments are contemporary to your generation. Do not get left behind and learn everything that comes your way.

2) Protect your password—Keep your password a secret. Do not use obvious passwords like your name or date of birth, but keep something abstract and keep changing them without forgetting.

3) Think before you post—Whatever you post online, whatever websites you visit, they get easily observed by someone who wants to. So beware about what you post.

4) Do not open spam mail—Mails announcing that you have won a lottery or an attorney announcing that you are the sole benefactor of your distant uncle who died in Timbuktu, or a hapless damsel seeking your help with her business are all traps set for the vulnerable.

5) Honey traps—Good looking profiles of young opposite gender people sending you request for friendship, offering you romantic solutions for combating loneliness and asking your email ID or WhatsApp number are all cheap traps for the vulnerable. Do not visit shady websites because someone is watching you.

6) Fraudulent Shopping sites—Some online shopping sites apparently offer to sell some stuff at a throwaway prices or offer free deals which sound too good to be true. They track your credit card payment details and may cause extensive damage to into your bank account.

7) Fake Government officer—Beware of emails from fake Government officials or tax officials. Never respond to such mails.

8) Do not install random software—There might be pop ups inviting you to download certain software which will supposedly do amazing things for you. Never touch them. They can fish out your important data.

9) Free Wi-Fi—Never connect your phone or laptop to free Wi-Fi. Cyber criminals are on the prowl everywhere.

10) Be a S.M.A.R.T. senior
    Stay safe—Do not share personal information
    Meet—Do not meet / date strangers online
    Accept—Do not accept suspicious files
    Reliable—Check if information is reliable
    Tell—Tell someone if you feel insecure about something

In this chapter, we learned how to beware of imposters and fraudsters. The cyber world appears to be confidential, but it is in fact more transparent and open than we think. In the next chapter we shall explore the efficacy of various age-reversing formulae.

Key takeaways:

1. *Guard your passwords with your life.*

2. *Maintain your privacy of information.*

3. *Whatever sounds too good to be true is often not true at all.*

Part 4: Aging Gracefully

Chapter 9: REVERSE AGING

Can medical science stop aging?

What secrets have our scientists discovered about reverse aging technology?

Back in the 1800s, average human lifespan was 40, but now people live twice that long. People died young because of lack of medical care, frequent childbirth among women, combat & hunting among men and now, with unchecked pandemic precaution. With medical science, it's easy to assume that our lifespan has soared over the last century and a half. However, with increasing age, the risk of chronic disease and disability have risen.

The goal is to use preventive measures to target aging, which is the major risk factor for a wide variety of diseases and disabilities, instead of treating one disease at a time, which is very costly. A future model from the Office of Budget Responsibility projected an increase in NHS expenditure of £42 million year-on-year until 2031 because of the aging population.

Reverse aging technology would increase not only lifespan, but health-span, which is the period of our life for which we are healthy, happy, and productive. It would continually restore vitality and bodily function by eliminating the damage that is compulsorily caused by the aging processes.

Older people are more susceptible to chronic diseases, that is responsible for primary causes of death around the world. Slowing down the aging process can help prevent diseases because it lowers the risk of conditions like diabetes, cardiovascular disease, strokes, Alzheimers, Parkinsons and Malignancy.

An aging population puts a burden on the economy. The productivity of old people decreases and their dependence on the health service increases. Becoming older increases the vulnerability of getting serious diseases like Alzheimers and Parkinsons that reduce the quality of life and are expensive and bothersome to treat.

What if reversing age was likely? Treating individual conditions in their old age is expensive, but to slow down aging to keep their youth for longer is more sensible. With sustained youthfulness, people will be stronger and less prone to illness.

Reverse aging technology has the potential to benefit for human longevity and health. The longer a person can live healthily, happily and more productive, the better it is for society too, because it could relieve the burden on the country's economy and health services.

Can they reverse aging?

It is important to understand the human aging timeline before analyzing the possibility that scientists could reverse the aging process. The cells in the body undergo several metabolic reactions relentlessly. Although unavoidable, they release toxic metabolites that accumulate, until eventually, they contribute to a weakening of the cells till they perish.

Also, our genes and the environment in which we live in also affect the human aging timeline. Aging is a balance between birth of new cells vs their rate of death, repair of cells through nutrition and sleep, our genetic codes, and the environment. 25% cause of longevity may get attributed to your genes, affecting cell metabolism and supporting processes which slow down aging, but there are many other factors which contribute to average life expectancy. For example, smoking can reduce lifespan, whereas mindful eating and regular exercise may extend it.

Reverse aging technology

They have shown experiments and trials on reversing the aging process to be possible using human stem cells and simple organisms, but the possibility to reverse ageing in humans is still a hype.

Researchers have been experimenting on simpler organisms like mice, to understand impact of interventions such as intermittent fasting and targeting the molecular proteins associated with the aging process may provide hints for humans too.

In one study, researchers connected the circulatory systems of an aged mouse with a young mouse and discovered that the young mouse began aging while the old mouse became younger, as their old and young blood mixed.

However, it is still too early to expect for reverse aging technology, Humans are complex beings, so therapies which show a possibility in mice may not work for us.

As of now, your best bet currently is a DNA health test, like the one by U.K. company Atlas Biomed, that tests your potential risk for diseases and provides you with personalized tips to help prevent them so you may live longer and healthier.

Impact of lifestyle on aging

There are some changes you can implement into your lifestyle to reverse ageing by improving your health and lowering your risk of untimely death from common but preventable diseases. To begin with, take a health DNA test to get recommendations for a proper lifestyle.

Moderate exercise is important, and research shows it has major benefits that contribute for your longevity too. A study comparing older adults who had exercised for most part of their lives with individuals who didn't exercise, showed that the regular exercisers had fewer problems related to reduced muscle mass and loss of strength. Also, cholesterol and body fat levels amongst this control group didn't increase with aging, highlighting the importance of physical activity throughout life, and their testosterone levels remained high into older age. The study also showed that exercise had a greater impact on the immune systems of older adults. Research saw these adults to be producing more T-cells, a type of immune cell, as younger, healthy people — meaning their bodies are better prepared to ward off illnesses.

The impact of diet on reverse aging

Eating mindfully and eating lesser than your belly's capacity has shown to have a positive impact on mice, primates, and humans. Ideally, one should eat 80% of one's capacity to eat. The benefits include a reduced risk of heart disease, diabetes, and stroke with little effect on factors such as mood, sleep quality, and libido.

In my observation with the health of myself and family, there are two prime factors for health. One is the digestive system, and the other is psychological balance. Stress and anxiety triggers acidity. Acidity boosts up bad cholesterol, which is an enzyme that increases because of prolonged acidity. Cholesterol is responsible for various cardio-vascular and other diseases. Treating those with statins not only kills your libido but also wrenches your liver, forcing it to over-perform. The overall health deteriorates, which further adds to stress and anxiety. Overuse of antacids have other disastrous effects. Hence you have to work upon keeping these two primary wheels healthy. The digestive system and the psychology.

However, reducing calorie intake is difficult for people who have to perform manual work, and that's where intermittent fasting helps. It's an eating pattern which, unlike dieting, doesn't tell you which foods to eat, but when you should eat them.

They apply intermittent fasting in various ways by different diet experts. Some of them are:

1. Random fasting—In this method there is no pattern of fasting, but you eat only when you are hungry and skip meals when you are not hungry.

2. Raw food + one meal diet—In this method, you eat only fresh fruits and raw vegetables / salad sans dressing throughout the day, and then have one major meal of cooked food (preferably

balanced diet) before sunset. After that, you eat nothing.

3. 8:16 method—In this method you eat the first meal at noon and last meal at 8 p.m. Thereafter you fast overnight till next noon.

4. Fast diet method—In this method, you partially fast for two days in a week. It is like you eat today normally, then fast by taking 25% of normal calorie intake, and then eat normally for two days, and then fast again. People observe completely fast on those two days in this same method, consuming no calories.

5. Alternate days fasting—In this method you eat normally one day and fast the next day or maybe have a tiny low calorie meal. So you eat and fast on alternate days.

Diets are fads that keep coming around in novel forms, but their efficacy is yet to get proven scientifically.

The impact of nootropic supplements

Nootropics are natural supplements that have a positive effect on brain function in healthy people. Some of these can boost memory, motivation, creativity, alertness and general cognitive function. Nootropics may also reduce age-related declines in brain function.

1. **Vitamin B6 & Phosphorous** - Studies show that students who ate bananas could learn more efficiently and improve their scores in exams. They contain phosphorus, which builds the brain and also contain vitamin B6, which promotes the production of serotonin, norepinephrine and dopamine to support concentration.

2. **Fish Oils** - Fish oil supplements are a rich source of Docosahexaenoic acid (DHA) and Eicosapentaenoic acid (EPA), two types of omega-3 fatty acids. They have linked these fatty acids with many health benefits, including improved brain health. If you do not eat fish, then consider a capsule containing fish oil.

3. Resveratrol - Resveratrol is an antioxidant that's found in the skin of purple and red fruits like grapes, raspberries and blueberries. It's also found in red wine, chocolate and peanuts but in very low concentration. For the required amount of dosage, it's recommended that resveratrol supplements could prevent the deterioration of the hippocampus, an important part of the brain associated with memory. In animals, it has shown that resveratrol supplements improve memory and brain function. It's not yet clear if the treatment has the same effects on people.

4. Caffeine - Caffeine is a natural stimulant that can improve your brain function and make you feel more energized and alert. It is a natural stimulant most commonly found in tea, coffee and dark chocolate. In fact, studies have shown that caffeine can make you feel more energized and improve your memory, reaction times and general brain function.

5. Phosphatidylserine- phosphatidylserine supplements could improve your thinking skills and memory. They could also help combat the decline in brain function as you age. However, further study is required to confirm its benefits.

6. Acetyl-L-Carnitine - Acetyl-L-carnitine could be helpful for treating a loss of brain function in the elderly and people with mental disorders such as dementia or Alzheimer's. Its effects on healthy people are unknown. Acetyl-L-carnitine is an amino acid produced naturally in your body and can be taken as vitamin supplements. It plays an important role in your metabolism, particularly in energy production.

7. Ginkgo Biloba - Ginkgo biloba may help improve your short-term memory and thinking skills. It may also protect you from age-related decline in brain function. However, results are inconsistent. It's a herbal supplement derived from the *Ginkgo biloba* tree. It's an incredibly popular supplement many people take to boost

their brain power by increasing blood flow to the brain and is claimed to improve brain functions like focus and memory.

8. Creatine - Taking creatine supplements could help improve memory and thinking skills in vegetarian people who don't eat meat. However, check out your renal profile because this may spike up your uric acid.

9. Bacopa Monnieri - Bacopa monnieri has shown to improve memory and thinking skills in healthy people and in those with a decline in brain function.

10. Rhodiola Rosea - Rhodiola rosea may help improve thinking skills by reducing fatigue. However, more research is required before scientists can be certain of its effects. It is a supplement derived from the herb *Rhodiola rosea*, which is often used in Chinese medicine to promote well-being and healthy brain function. It helps improve mental processing by reducing fatigue.

11. S-Adenosyl methionine - S-Adenosyl methionine (SAMe) is a substance that occurs naturally in your body. It's used in chemical reactions to make and break down important compounds like proteins, fats and hormones. SAMe could be useful for improving brain

function in people with depression. There is no evidence it has this effect on healthy people.

Are we close to reverse aging?

Reverse aging technology is still wishful desire, even though clinical trials are underway involving regenerative stem cell therapy for heart diseases. Even then, there are concerns that reversing aging in cells could lead to the uncontrollable multiplication of cells, resulting in cancer.

However, there are certain aspects of your own life that can help to increase your lifespan, which you can take control of by yourself. Lead a healthy lifestyle with plenty of exercise/ physical activity, a healthy diet, good sleep, and a happy mind can all go a long way to increase your abilities and health long into old age.

Imagine if your life is like a bicycle, then the front wheel is your mental happiness and rear wheel is a nourished body with the body frame and pedals as a moderate exercise that connects the body and mind together. There are many proven ways that can help you increase your lifespan by staying healthy well into old age, even if it doesn't mean reversing your biological age.

In this chapter we learned about various supplements commonly used for age reversing. Their efficacy is yet to get certified scientifically.

We shall read about the need for maturing up with age in the next chapter. We shall learn how to grow up mindfully and accept the aging process and its consequences.

Key takeaways:

1. *There are various supplements that claim age reversal.*

2. *These supplements have delivered random results and hopes.*

3. *Their efficacy is yet to get proven scientifically.*

Chapter 10: THE SECRET OF JAPANESE LONGEVITY

"Wrinkles should merely indicate, where smiles have been."—Mark Twain.

In a comparison of mortality statistics among various developed countries around the world, Japan has the longest average life expectancy, primarily because of remarkably low mortality rates from heart diseases and cancer.

A healthy diet, regular physical activity, extended work years and aggressive governmental initiatives, have helped with longevity in the Japanese. Their life expectancy is the highest in the world at 87.32 years for women and 81.25 years for men. In 2019, the number of Japanese aged 90 reached 2.31 million, including over 71,000 centenarians.

Here are 7 tips to gain longevity, like the Japanese.

Diet

The Japanese diet is a perfect example of Greek physician Hippocrates. He said, "May your food be your medicine, and your medicine be your food," which is a major reason for their long lifespans. Their diet is lean and balanced, with staple foods like omega-rich fish, rice, whole grains, tofu, fermented soy, miso, seaweed and plenty of vegetables. All these foods ensure adequate phytochemicals, vitamins and minerals. They are low in saturated fats and sugars and rich in vitamins and minerals that reduce the risk of cancers and heart disease.

Cooking Method

The typical Japanese cuisine involves a lot of steaming, fermenting, slow-cooking, pan grilling and stir-frying, which conserves the maximum nutrients in the food. They eat fresh food within a couple of hours after cooking. They don't have a fridge stashed with tinned foods to get microwaved and eaten whenever hungry. Eating fresh food gives a lot more nutrition and energy.

Eating Manners

They prepare small dishes, their portions are small and they eat with chopsticks. They never bite big mouthfuls and they chew slowly and mindfully. Their dinner time is quite ceremonial, with family sitting together and eating in total silence without watching TV or mobile screens during meals. They essentially begin every meal with a bowl of soup, so they never eat too much at a time.

Genetic Advantage

While things like good healthcare and a great diet have helped the Japanese to increase their lifespan, studies suggest they may have a genetic advantage.

DNA 5178 and ND2-237 are two specific genes which play a potential role in extending life by preventing the onset of some diseases. DNA 5178 helps people resist adult-onset diseases like type 2 diabetes, strokes and heart attacks. ND2-237 Met genotype also helps with resistance to cerebrovascular and cardiovascular diseases. Japanese people are more likely to have these genes.

Tea Culture

Sipping green tea frequently throughout the day is a Japanese culture that goes a long way in fighting diseases because of its anti-bacterial properties. Matcha tea, in particular, is beneficial for the body. They hardly drink iced water like the western world. They drop a 'tea coin' in a tall glass and keep pouring boiling water and sip while absorbing its warmth through their palms. Tea coins are green tea leaves woven in bamboo strips and crafted like a porous disk. Drinking warm water has various health benefits, including fighting obesity.

Excellent Healthcare

The long lifespan of the Japanese is also because of their excellent health care. Japan's health care system is one of the best in the world (ranked 4th by Bloomberg Efficient Health Care). Since the 1960s, the government has paid 70 per-cent of all health procedures and up to 90 per-cent for low-income citizens. They also have advanced medical knowledge and equipment, making Japan the ideal place to get old. The government has introduced many preventative measures to care for its citizens, such as health screenings in schools and workplaces. Along with government initiatives, proper health care is part of Japanese culture. Japanese citizens visit the doctor an average of 13 times a year for check-ups. This means that illnesses are more likely to get detected early.

Elder Care

It is Japanese tradition for people to respect and care for elderly family members rather than sending them to care homes. The psychological benefits of living with your family in old age means that people are happier and live longer.

Key takeaways:

1. The world can learn from the Japanese about how to live longer.

2. The Japanese live not only longer but healthier too.

3. Learn 7 ways to increase longevity like the Japanese.

Chapter 11: AGE-ing To SAGE-ing

"The Sky Gets Dark, Slowly," a novel by Zhou Daxin, Mao Dun literary prize winner is a sensitive exploration of old age and the complex, hidden emotional worlds of the elderly in a rapidly ageing population.

In it he composes, many elders talk like they know it all, yet about old age they are as oblivious as kids. Many elders get totally surprised for what they are to confront regarding getting old and the path that lays in front of them.

By the time an individual turns 60 years of age, as they age, until all the lights go out, the sky gets darker, there are a few circumstances to remember, so you will get prepared for what is coming, and you won't fret.

1. The individuals close by will just keep on becoming more modest. Individuals in your parents' and grandparents' age have totally left, while many friends will progressively think that it's harder to take care of themselves, and the more youthful kin will all be occupied with their own lives. Even your better half or spouse may withdraw sooner than you, or than you would expect, and what may then come are long stretches of solitude. You should figure out how to live alone, and to appreciate and grasp isolation.

2. Society will mind lesser for you. Regardless of how heavenly your past vocation was or how popular you were, ageing will consistently change you into a common old man / woman. The spotlight no longer radiates on you, and you need to figure out how to fight with standing unobtrusively in one corner, to respect

and like the commotion and perspectives that come after you, and defeat the desire to be jealous or protest.

3. The path ahead will be rough and brimming with precarity. Breaks, cardio-vascular blockages, cerebrum decay, malignancy, disease... these are potential visitors that could visit you any time, and you would not have the option to dismiss them. You should live with ailment and illnesses, to see them as companions, even; don't fantasize about steady and calm days with no difficulty in your body. Keeping an inspirational mindset and get proper, sufficient exercise is your obligation, and you need to urge yourself to keep at it reliably.

4. Plan for bed-ridden life, a re-visitation of the baby state. Our moms welcomed us into this world on a bed, and after an excursion of exciting bends in the road and a daily existence of battle, we re-visit our beginning stage, the bed, and to the condition of being taken care of by others. The solitary contrast being the place where we once had our moms to really focus on us; when we get ready to leave, we might not have our kinfolk to care for us. Regardless of whether we have family, their consideration may never match that of your mother's; you will get actually focused on by nursing staff who bear zero connection to you, wearing grins on their faces, all while conveying exhaustion and fatigue in their souls. Lay still and don't be troublesome; make sure to `be appreciative.

5. There will be many deceivers and con artists en route. A significant number of them realize that the old people have a lifetime of savings, and will interminably consider approaches to swindle them of their cash: through trick calls, instant messages, mail, super food and supplement samples, get rich quick schemes, items for longevity and age reversal... all they need is to rob all the cash from you. Be careful, and be cautious, hold

your cash near you. A dumb person can't help but get swindled, so spend your pennies wisely.

Before the sky gets dark, the last stretches of life's excursion will continuously get dimmer and dimmer; normally, it will be more diligently to see the way forward that you are stepping towards, and it will be more enthusiastically to continue to go ahead. After turning 60, it would do us all well to recognize the truth about existence, to treasure what we have, to appreciate life while we can, and to not interpretation of society's inconveniences or your kids' and grandkids' undertakings on for yourself. Stay humble, don't act predominant because of your own age and patronize others; this will hurt yourself as much as it will hurt others. As we get older, all the better should we have the option to comprehend what respect is and what it means. In these later days of your lives, you need to comprehend what it implies, to relinquish your connections, to intellectually set yourself up. The method of nature is the lifestyle; go with its stream and live with composure.

Test Your Maturity Level

Are you matured? Have you wondered if you have matured? What is Maturity?

Maturity is a state of mind which is in awareness to realize what is happening around, and you can understand the rationale behind things that are happening. Thus, if you can absorb the pressures and excitement of the situations so you are neither too elated nor too depressed by the situations and their outcome.

You would know that your gray matter has gained wisdom if you observe most of the following traits in you.

1. You are a listener

When you listen, just listen. Are you listening to understand someone's perspective, or are you listening just to answer back? Everyone loves a good listener because most people have the urge to speak more and listen less. Also, are you just hearing or listening objectively? If you are listening, then you are hearing with interest, purpose and intent to understand what is being said. Wisdom is in knowing, learning, understanding and analyzing.

2. You would rather accommodate than argue

A mature person would know that he/she is right yet let go of an argument. He/she understands that winning the argument is not as important as holding on to the relationship. You are allowing the other person to keep his/her dignity and providing him/her space and time to realize after sometime and understand that you were right. If the other person eventually realizes that, then your prestige and command shall increase in his/her eyes.

3. You are eager to take responsibility

To begin with, you take responsibility for your own actions and needs. You do not depend on other people for everything. The sense of responsibility grows in you spatially. Your domain of inclusiveness extends over your family, friends, society, communities and the nation. You empathize with issues concerning entire humanity and the eco-system. You realize you inherited a beautiful world and you must give it back to the next generation as is if not with some improvement.

4. You get along well with everyone

A wise person can get along well with people of all age groups, gender, level of education and intellect and their economic status. You have risen above the differences that divide humans into various compartmentalized segments. You can see the inner divinity in every human and can relate yourself with everyone.

5. You are at peace with yourself

Does sunshine brighten up your day? Does rain water down your enthusiasm? Do you feel that the dark winters are gloomy? A wise person would feel comfortable in all seasons and weather. To him/her, it is just nature at its work. You are as happy in the mountains as by the seashore. You admire the sand dunes as much as the lush green forests. You do not get perturbed by changes. You understand nothing remains static. Everything changes according to its cyclical nature. You are mindful that the best things in this universe are happening silently with minimum efforts and there is no point in chasing something too hard.

6. You can prioritize

You have realized that wants and needs are unlimited and resources are only as many. You have learned to prioritize. For accommodating someone else's priority over your own, you do not hesitate. You know it is important to take care of yourself and hence you always attend to your body, mind and soul. Also, you take care of others around you because you understand the value of care.

7. You have gained wise habits

You have gained wise habits like reading, meditation, exercise, mindful eating, financial planning and balancing our life. You are an active and sociable person. You take up causes on behalf of people and you are capable to guide. The seeds of learning that you have gathered in your life, you sow them back and give them the energy of the environment to multiply and enhance.

8. You do not fear death

You know that when a leaf withers away, there is another fresh leaf sprouting at the node to take its place. You understand that excessive longevity or immortality can do more harm than good. Also, you realize that as the body grows; it accumulates certain level of toxicity which causes aging, and sometimes death salvages the person from the pains of these toxins. You can see ultimate liberation through death. As a responsible person, you have left none critical responsibility unfinished and you are ready for the onward journey. You can detach yourself from the worldliness and keep performing your duty while you are alive without being flustered about its consequence. You understand how death enables your inner energy to mingle with the universal source of energy and how it can transcend into another wavelength.

9. You do not carry an emotional baggage

You know that while departing from this life, you shall not be able to carry anything with you. During the last moments, one might feel the heaviness of emotional baggage. Do you still bear a grudge? Have you unburdened yourself by forgiving and moving on? Wise people never carry this load till the end. They are mindful of their karma because they know their actions could benefit or hurt someone else. They do their best to ensure their action should hurt that nobody.

10. Your happiness lies within you

You have become the source of your own happiness. You are not dependent on the occurrence of an event or gaining something materially to become happy because you have realized that if the source of happiness is external, then the state of happiness is temporary because once you lose that material object, you will lose the happiness as well. Your happiness wells out from within you like a spring. Happiness becomes your natural state of mind, and your state of exuberance easily gets rubbed on to the others as well. You always wear a smile and even if there is a moment of frown, you know how to turn it upside down. Adult education advisor Elizabeth Lesser said: *"It's like you trade the virility of the body for the agility of the spirit."*

11. You seek the signs of maturity

You seek signs of maturity, and that is one reason you chose to read this book. This action itself shows you are serious about being mature. Maturity brings with it responsibility. With responsibility comes sensibility. Sensibility leads to confidence. So move with confidence to show the world you have now matured.

"My physical body may be less efficient and less beautiful in old age. But God has given me an enormous compensation: my mind is richer, my Soul is broader and my wisdom is at a peak. I am so happy with the riches of my advanced peak age that, contrary to Faust, I would not wish to return to youth." - Robert Muller [Jury Counsel]

In this chapter we learned how to become mature to realize the condition that everyone is gradually aging and hence it is important to gain maturity to accept yourself with changed circumstances. We also carried out a test to measure our maturity level. Further, we shall arrive at the conclusion to this narrative.

> ### *Key takeaways:*
>
> 1. Zhou Daxin in his book The Sky Gets Dark has stated four imperative circumstances upon aging.
>
> 2. We have tested our maturity level by ticking off eleven signs of maturity.
>
> 3. Aging is mandatory, growing-up is a choice.

Chapter 12: The Conclusion

In the Indian system of social science, it categorizes the lifespan of a human into four stages.

1. Brahmacharya ashram—Celibacy stage
2. Grishasta ashram–Family stage
3. Vanprastha ashram—Detachment stage
4. Sanyas ashram—Renunciation stage

During the first quarter of the life, it requires a person to maintain celibacy and focus on learning and gaining skills. The education system in those days was of the Gurukul system. This is like university hostel where students stay with their teacher and learn. It gave them knowledge as per with their aptitude and ability.

The second quarter was for family life. In this phase people married and beget children. They earned money according to their knowledge and skills. They remained fully devoted to their business & profession and family.

In the third stage, people could see the dusk of their lives. They passed on their active roles to their next generation and took up advisory roles. They followed their own pursuit of self-actualization through yoga, meditation, religious activities, shaping their grandchildren with social and moral values and gradually detaching themselves from all kinds of active roles.

The last stage was harsh. Old people actually left their homes and ventures out in the forests. They either camped into some hermitage awaiting death or perish in absence of basic amenities, or got killed by wild animals. The aim was to keep the society free of the old and dying population. In today's modern world it should translate as giving up self-centric ways, accepting your physical and mental limitations, not interfering or manipulating into the affairs of family and business and keep peace within self.

Reality check

At large, the society is not functioning in the manner it should. In their student days, people are not aspiring to learn sincerely and become the best. There is a lot of scope for distraction and they succumb to mediocrity. Having failed to make a solid base in the initial phase of life, they make a meek start in their next stage of life for their career and family. If the education and skills remained inept, it becomes hard to make a suitable career and even harder to raise a family. Such people cannot move up to the stage of self-actualization, and their life remains a struggle within existential crisis. Finally, they usher into prolonged sickness and old age and perish after a miserable phase of battling with various diseases.

You can take out an old engine from your garage, tinker it, oil it and try to make it run. Will you be able to run it efficiently? You have an old engine in a running condition, regularly oiled and serviced and used efficiently. Which of these two machines do you think would serve you more efficiently? Obviously it is the latter which got serviced regularly. Likewise, is the functioning of our body. We do not wake up after 60 to prime up our rusty old engine. We have to keep ourselves primed up all our life so we do not end up like a rusted tin-box in the junkyard. That is why at the outset I mentioned, this book is not only for the old but also for the young people who will become old someday. I hope this book has enabled you to set priorities in life.

While writing this book, I have maintained my stance that you have to keep the right direction and life and make the right choices in every stage of your life. Your actions for today will affect your future life ahead.

I was discussing my thoughts with several of my friends who are middle-aged and every discussion lead to understanding a new perspective about the challenges faced during aging.

One such interesting conversation I had was with Father George Mary Claret. He is a catholic priest and a dear friend. He works with the communities and gets first hand interaction with several people who are young or old, rich or poor, and he listens to their problems and tries to suggest solutions to help them. Here is what he had to say.

People are without fire. They are mostly purposeless in life. Most people have misplaced their thoughts and have made raising their children as the sole purpose of their lives. They just lived for their children and had no life of their own. Once their children grow up and move out of the house, it leaves them with no other purpose in life than to live in despair and wait for death. It is not just about the old people who are waiting to die. Even as children, they are mostly living with no purposefulness. Further, even as young people, they are mostly like floating driftwood. They may get driven by some random undercurrent, but they are seldom self-propelling. People are living between B to D without considering C. B is birth and D is death. In between C means choices. Unfortunately, people are just making it from birth to death without making the choices in their life.

In this book we have learned that life has a different meaning for every person from his/her own perspective. Therefore, each person has to define his/her own life. The world appears to be entirely different from my perspective than yours, and you and I would see it differently. For each one of you, the center of your universe is just you, and everything that you can experience is around you. For this reason, you are entirely responsible for your own life. Your life shall be like how you make it. Life is a simple process. We were born without our asking and got raised by our mother in her way. Once we grow up to be on our own, it's all about our experiences and actions. The experiences we go through in life got received through our sensory organs and got accumulated into our memory bank. What we reflect upon is a recall of our memories. It is upon us to choose what sort of memories we wish to gather for ourselves.

An ECG Electrocardiogram of a living person has waves depicting the heartbeat. The graph is as a line fluctuating above and below the baseline.

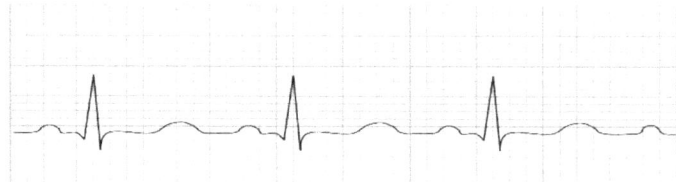

Whereas the ECG of a lifeless person shall be in a straight line. Do not expect a straight line always. Life is not a straight line, but a series of ups and down. Life will throw situations and circumstances at our face. The onus lies on us to decide how we tackle those, how we change the outcome of our experiences and what sort of memories we wish to collect for ourselves. Our experiences will depend on the choices we make instead of the intensity of the circumstances alone.

The later phases of life will differ from the first two phases, but we have to learn to accept the change. We have to make our choices mindfully so we can have the desired experiences. We have to filter our memory to keep those experiences we cherish.

The time clock shall continue ticking. Everyone gets an equal measure of time and almost a similar measure of abilities to perform. Yet some people have a more meaningful life than others because they made their choices rightly.

While crossing one milestone after the other in your life, do not lose focus on the purpose of your life. A life with no purpose becomes difficult to carry. Hence, always try to have some purpose in your life. Continue to set small goals and achieve them. Keep your mind and body active. After achieving one small goal, set another one slightly larger than previously.

Instead of lamenting about what you do not have or what you cannot, be grateful to what you have and what you still can. Instead of bearing grudges, forgive and forget and jettison your emotional baggage. Do not focus on your pains and miseries alone, but channelize your remaining strength.

To conclude in the words of an American teacher of yoga and meditation, Rod Stryker, *"Your long-term happiness and fulfillment depend on your ability to fulfill your soul's unique purpose and to fill the place in the world that only you can fill, making the contribution that only you can make."*

ONE MOMENT PLEASE

I thank you with deep gratitude for having read this book till the end. You could have read any other book, but you chose this one and I sincerely hope this was worth your time.

I hope you found practical solutions to your questions about aging, and if you liked my work, I request you to please spend a few moments to follow through this link and post a feedback on Amazon. Please click here.

If you have any suggestions or questions about this book, you can reach me through support@mylifesutra.com or leave a comment on www.mylifesutra.net. Follow me on my Author Central page on Amazon through Click to follow to stay in touch with my next books.

Please watch out for my other publications on Amazon Central. I shall continue to serve you with my writing. Hope to stay connected.

GRATITUDE

I owe this book to my aged parents and grandparents, whose experiences in life gave me an opportunity to learn how to shape my future.

I bow to my parents, elders, Gurus, teachers, mentors, guides, friends, prominent personalities—my role models, who have helped shape me as the individual I am; and for the insights I have gained from them about life, that have enabled me to write.

I express deep gratitude to my readers who showered their love and appreciation for my debut book "THE SECRETS TO A MAGICAL LIFE" which became Amazon#1 International Bestseller within a month of its launch. Also grateful to my readers for their repeated love for my second book, "HOW TO GROW RICH AND BECOME WEALTHY." Their support and encouragement has given me the energy and inspiration to continue writing.

I am grateful to my dear friend and author-cum-graphics designer Ranjit Jose for crafting a beautiful book cover that caught your attention. Photographs Courtesy: 1. Nathan Dumlao, Brand Consultant and Content Creator, Los Angeles, USA. @Unsplash - Hour Glass 2. Jacob Rudge, Designer and founder of trade Happy. @Unsplash - Man in the Background

ABOUT THE AUTHOR

Vikram Khaitan is an author, mentor, creative and enthusiastic speaker, a seeker and philosopher who looks beyond the existing challenges to find solutions for the future. His keen sense of observation and comprehension of life makes him look at things differently.

He holds a niche in personal development. His works reflect his lucid writing and simple conversation skills with excerpts and interesting anecdotes from his personal experiences. He brings across solutions to help improve life, develop a positive attitude, enhance the thought process, improve career, money & finance, health, relationships and the mind. His books aim to be your path-finder for success in life.

He has also authored the Amazon#1 international bestseller, "The Secrets to a Magical Life." His second book also was a roaring success and is available on Amazon as. "How To Grow Rich And Become Wealthy."

Contact the author at www.mylifesutra.in and email support@mylifesutra.in

DISCLAIMER

The content of this book deals with various life skills which got widely accepted and followed across the world, including India. My perceptions and understanding may coincide with people who share common values with me or contradict with the beliefs of those who disagree with me. There is no intention to endorse someone else's learning as mine because I have sought my own truths and beliefs through my research, practice and experience. Also, I do not intend to hurt the sentiments of anyone, because this is my story as I perceive it to be and we all see the world from our own unique point of view.

MY PREVIOUS WORKS

My dear readers, you might have read my previous work titled as "***The Secrets To A Magical Life***"

Within three weeks of its release it became #1 International Bestseller in USA (Amazon.com), Canada (amazon.ca) and Australia (Amazon.com.au) and #1 Hot new release in U.K. (amazon.co.uk). The book has sold across nine countries across the globe.

Please click here to check it out today.

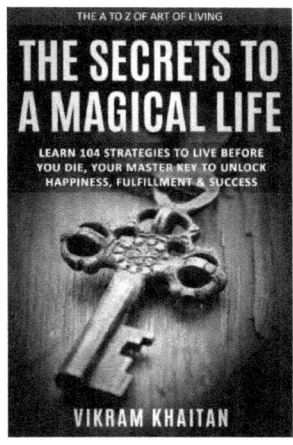

Here is what my readers said about this book:

1. "*I like how you use examples and illustrative stories to get teaching points across. Makes me think of the way Dr. Srikumar Rao also teaches and writes.*" - Ms. Jacqueline Fox–MS-Program Manager, The Rao Institute (via Gmail)

2. *"Amazing insights into how to experience magical life. It focuses on how we can improve our lives and be joyful."*—Vijay Elhence

3. *"Upon reading this book, I can surely say it's Inspiring, Interesting, allows you to do self-observance & self-improvement and many more.... Author has narrated life's event in very crisp manner that it becomes difficult to keep this book aside once you've started reading it. I loved it because I could link up many events of my life which got overlooked in today's competitive busy life..."* - Adv. Swapnil Modi.

4. *"Situations come in life when life looks like a mess. Feeling comes like we are heading for nowhere everything goes off color. Whenever anyone comes to face such a situation, finding no outlet for worries to drain out, then this book can give you some simple solutions to make yourself feel special once again. For many, this book can be a ray of hope and a true game changer. Writer deserves a big thank for bringing such a meaningful content in such simple words."*—Vijay Bisht

5. *"Excellent book. Chapters are short and arranged beautifully. Many incidents in the book are really eye openers. The book gave me a new perspective about life. There are so many simple but practical exercises mentioned in the book."*- Sujith George

6. *"Powerful Life Mantra! Superb ideas to follow and implement to achieve success in life. The language of the book is simple, with powerful life mantras for success. This book will help you train your mind and body to develop the strength of healthy intelligence and enable you to deal with all situations. Highly recommended!"*—Ajit Jha

7. *"A very inspiring and well-written book. The book exudes positivity and the hacks to the Magical life are doable for most of us. The examples illustrated are simple and very apt quotes to support... truly Magical."*—Dr. Madhavan

8. *"Amazing reading experience, you won't put this book down - and it's full of magical ideas - a must read for one and all! Highly recommended!"*—Dr. Anand Ahuja

9. *"The perfect guide for improving your life quality. The book grooves effectively into the real insights of life, using every small to big example, the author has described the hacks for a brighter life ahead. It is full of positivity and an amazing self-help guide to unleash true potentials."*—Ayshi Ganguly

Also, read my second craft, "**How To Grow Rich And Become Wealthy.**" Please click here to check it out today.

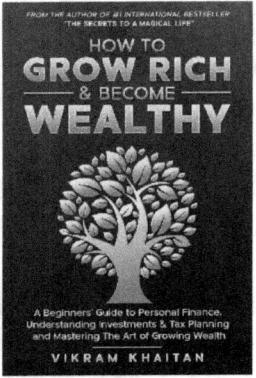

Here is what my readers said about this book:

1. *"A great overview that makes it easy to take action. It's entertaining and takes you step by step, at your own pace, into the complex world of decisions and priorities to make. I look forward to his next book. Great work!"*-Dan Agervig Hansen.

2. *"Wealth is the yardstick to know how well one is using one's abilities. Many of the richest persons in the modern era were economically poor. They harnessed the means and found the right mentors to become what they are today. Vikram Khaitan is such a mentor. Through this simple yet very informative and practical book, he guides one by the hand as I felt. It is must read for all age groups as there is no age bar for growth."*-Fr.C. George Mary Claret.

3. *"The cover itself sets the tone that this book is about creating wealth for yourself as you grow. A very useful book for all those looking for understanding the art of saving from an early age. The suggestions are very doable and help the reader get conscious about the habit of saving for your dusk years. I recommend this book to the readers of all ages to stay happy in your retirement. Great reading."*-Virendra Kashyap.

4. *"Personal finance is a field about which most of us do not know! In this book, the author takes the reader through a journey towards financial freedom in a step-by-step manner, ensuring none of the important aspect gets missed out. The book develops both the MIND-SET and the SKILL-SET, which are required to grow rich and wealthy. There is a stark difference between being RICH and being WEALTHY, immerse yourself in this piece of wisdom to unearth the recipe."*-Santosh Singh.

5. *"An uninterrupted dialogue with every professional help to manage and grow your finances. A guide with the detailing of book-keeping and providing even formats along with the information that how markets behave is just amazing. A must have for all households."*-Anupama Rawat.

REFERENCES

I acknowledge the following publications I have used for carrying out my research for supporting the contents of my book.

1. News on Israeli research on age reversal - https://www.dnaindia.com/health/news-dna-special-are-we-close-to-reversing-biological-ageing-process-2858115

2. Story of Yayati - https://www.newindianexpress.com/opinions/2017/feb/18/why-is-king-yayati-so-important-1571786.html#:~:text=By%20Tanuj%20Solanki-,A%20fter%20losing%20his%20youth%20due%20to%20a%20curse%20from,their%20youth%20to%20their%20father.

   https://www.speakingtree.in/blog/the-story-of-yayati

   https://en.wikipedia.org/wiki/Yayati

3. Quotes - https://landmarkseniorliving.com/101-timeless-quotes-about-aging/

   https://www.smartliving365.com/50-best-positive-aging-quotes-find/

   https://www.positivityblog.com/friendship-quotes/

4. W.H.O. response - https://www.who.int/news-room/fact-sheets/detail/ageing-and-health#:~:text=Common%20conditions%20in%20older%20age,conditions%20at%20the%20same%20time.

5. Immunity Builders - https://www.healthline.com/nutrition/how-to-boost-immune-health#1.-Get-enough-sleep

6. https://www.realbuzz.com/articles-interests/health/article/tips-to-help-you-stay-young/

7. Yoga benefits - https://www.artofliving.org/in-en/yoga/health-and-wellness/anti-aging-yoga

   https://www.india.com/lifestyle/anti-aging-yoga-exercises-these-5-yoga-exercises-will-make-you-look-younger-1923682/

8. Changes in body with ageing - https://www.merckmanuals.com/home/older-people%E2%80%99s-health-issues/the-aging-body/changes-in-the-body-with-aging?query=ear%20care%20for%20ageing

9. East vs West - http://www.1000ventures.com/business_guide/crosscuttings/cultures_east-west-phylosophy.html

10. Live your life - https://aging.com/the-way-of-living-being-happy-and-healthy-at-an-old-age/

11. Mental wellbeing - https://www.nia.nih.gov/health/depression-and-older-adults

12. Late bloomers stories - https://paulrohan.medium.com/ten-of-historys-greatest-late-bloomers-people-who-found-their-purpose-and-went-for-awe-6b733c6fa154

13. Reverse aging - https://atlasbiomed.com/blog/can-science-stop-aging-the-facts-on-age-reversal-technology/

14. https://www.healthline.com/nutrition/best-nootropic-brain-supplements

www.ingramcontent.com/pod-product-compliance
Lightning Source LLC
Chambersburg PA
CBHW071413210526
45465CB00001B/361